Before We Are Born

Basic Embryology and Birth Defects

Keith L. Moore, Ph.D., F.I.A.C.

Professor and Head, Department of Anatomy, Faculties
of Medicine and Dentistry, University of Manitoba, and
Consultant in Anatomy, Children's Centre, Winnipeg, Canada

WITH 228 DRAWINGS AND PHOTOGRAPHS, 15 IN COLOR

W. B. SAUNDERS COMPANY

Philadelphia · London · Toronto

W. B. Saunders Company: West Washington Square
Philadelphia, PA   19105

12 Dyott Street
London, WC1A   1DB

833 Oxford Street
Toronto, Ontario M8Z 5T9, Canada

The illustration on the front cover is a photograph of
an embryo of about thirty-eight days.

Before We Are Born   ISBN   0-7216-6450-4

Last digit is the print number: 9   8   7   6   5   4   3   2

TO THE WOMEN IN MY LIFE
my wife Marion and our four daughters
AND MY SON WARREN
*without whose interest and encouragement
this book would not have been written*

PREFACE

This relatively simple account of human development was written primarily for students in the allied health sciences, especially those in physical and occupational therapy, nursing, pharmacy and dental hygiene. It may be useful to medical and dental students wishing a concise account of clinically oriented embryology, especially in schools where the study of this subject has been severely curtailed. It will also be of interest to students in physical and health education, biology, psychology, home economics and art. Persons with a special interest in this fascinating subject should consult the author's book entitled "The Developing Human: Clinically Oriented Embryology" and other suggestions for additional reading listed at the back of the present book.

Each chapter, except the first one, is followed by a summary, but it must be realized that each chapter is itself only a summary of essential facts and concepts. The book is freely illustrated to help beginning students visualize developmental processes and to understand the basis of congenital malformations. Most illustrations are diagrammatic, some in color, and show successive stages of development, conveying ideas and processes as blackboard sketches do during lectures. The terminology is based mainly on the Nomina Embryologica adopted by the Ninth International Congress of Anatomists held at Leningrad in August, 1970.

Winnipeg, Canada   KEITH L. MOORE

ACKNOWLEDGMENTS

The author is greatly indebted to Mr. Glen Reid, Medical Illustrator, and to Mrs. Brenda Bell, Medical Photographer, for preparing the illustrations. Although acknowledgment has been given in the legends to the illustrations, I should like to express collectively my appreciation to the various authors and publishers who granted permission to use their photographs in this book. Of the many colleagues who helped in writing this book, I particularly wish to thank Dr. T.V.N. Persaud, Associate Professor of Anatomy, and Miss Jean Hay, Assistant Professor of Anatomy.

I am much obliged to Miss Barbara Waller and her associates for the secretarial work. I am also grateful to my wife, Marion, for her help and encouragement. I should also like to express my appreciation to Mr. Walter Bailey, Vice President, W. B. Saunders Company, Toronto, who encouraged me to write this book, and to Mr. John Dusseau, Vice President and Editor, whose advice and help were much appreciated.

K.L.M.

CONTENTS

1
INTRODUCTION

Human development begins when an ovum (egg) is fertilized by a sperm. Development is a process of change that transforms the fertilized ovum, which is a single cell called a *zygote*, into a multicellular human being.

STAGES OF DEVELOPMENT

Development is divided into *prenatal* and *postnatal* periods. Birth is a dramatic event during development, but important developmental changes occur after birth (e.g., the teeth and the female breasts). The developmental stages occurring before we are born are illustrated in the *Timetables of Human Prenatal Development* (Figs. 1–1 and 1–2). The following list explains the terms used in these timetables:

Zygote. This cell is the beginning of a human being. It results from the fertilization of an ovum (egg) by a sperm (spermatozoon).

Cleavage. Division or cleavage of the zygote by mitosis[1] forms daughter cells called *blastomeres*. The blastomeres become smaller and smaller at each succeeding division.

Morula. When 16 or so blastomeres have formed, the ball of cells is called a morula because it resembles a mulberry.

Blastocyst. After the morula passes through the uterine tube and into the uterus (see Chapter 3), a cavity forms in it. This converts the morula into a blastocyst.

Embryo. The cells which give rise to the embryo appear as an *inner cell mass.* The term embryo is not usually used until the *embryonic disc* forms (see Chapter 4). The *embryonic period* extends until about the end of the seventh week, by which time the beginnings of all major structures are present.

Fetus. After the embryonic period, the developing human is called a fetus. During the *fetal period* (eighth week to birth), many systems develop further. Although developmental changes are not so dramatic as those occurring during the embryonic period, they are very important.

Conceptus. This term is used when referring to the embryo (or fetus) and its membranes, i.e., the *products of conception.*

The Importance of Embryology

The study of prenatal stages of development, especially those occurring during the embryonic period, helps us to understand the normal relationships of body structures and the causes of congenital malformations. The embryo is extremely vulnerable during the first three months to radiation, viruses and certain drugs (see Chapter 9). The physician's knowledge of normal development and the causes of congenital malformations aids in giving the embryo the greatest possible chance of developing normally. Much of the modern practice of obstetrics involves what might be called "applied developmental biology."

The significance of embryology is readily apparent to pediatricians because many of their patients have disorders resulting from maldevelopment, e. g., spina bifida and congenital heart disease. Progress in surgery,

---

[1]A method of division of a cell by means of which two daughter cells receive identical complements of chromosomes. For details of this process, see a histology textbook.

(Text continued on page 6.)

TIMETABLE OF HUMAN PRENATAL DEVELOPMENT
1 to 6 weeks

PROLIFERATIVE PHASE

BEGINNING OF MATURATION OF FOLLICLE

MENSTRUAL PHASE

COMPLETION OF MATURATION OF FOLLICLE

CONTINUATION OF THE PROLIFERATIVE PHASE

SECRETORY PHASE OF MENSTRUAL CYCLE

day 1 of menses

ovulation

midcycle

ovum

1 fertilization	2 zygote divides	3 4 blastomeres	4 cleavage of zygote in uterine tube	5 section of
		morula		blastocyst
6 implantation begins	7 embryonic endoderm visible			

8 bilaminar disc	9 primitive yolk sac	10 implantation complete	11 Primitive placental circulation established.	12 extraembryonic mesoderm
amniotic cavity	lacunae appear	epithelium growing over surface defect		coelom
13 primary villi	14 dorsal aspect of embryo			
	prochordal plate / embryonic disc			

AGE (weeks) 1 2

2

Figure 1–1. *Continued on opposite page.*

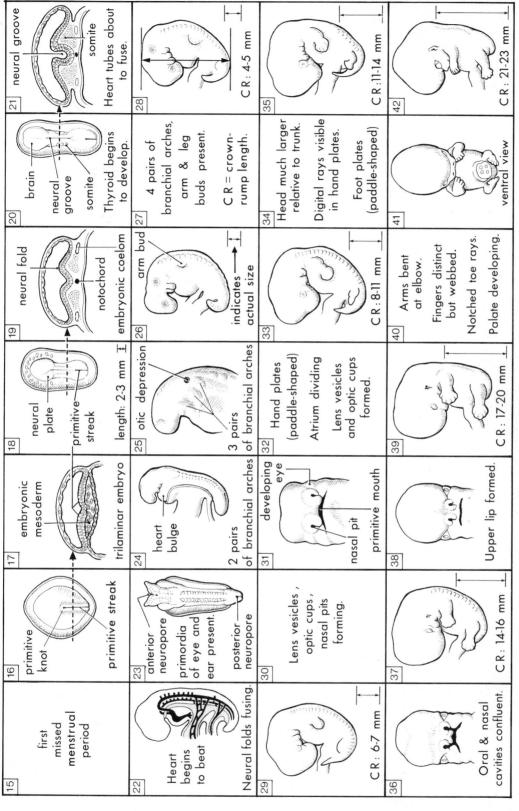

Figure 1–1. Maturation of a follicle containing a developing ovum (egg), ovulation and the menstrual cycle are illustrated. *Development begins at fertilization*, about 14 days after the onset of the last menstruation. Cleavage of the zygote in the uterine tube, implantation of the blastocyst and early development of the embryo are also shown.

TIMETABLE OF HUMAN PRENATAL DEVELOPMENT
7 to 38 weeks

43 CR: 22-24 mm.

44

45 CR: 25-27 mm.

46 Loss of villi Chorion laeve forms.

47 genital tubercle — urogenital membrane — anal membrane ♀ or ♂

48 Beginnings of all essential external & and internal structures are present.

49 CR: 31 mm

50 beginning of fetal period

51 Anal membrane perforated Urogenital membrane degenerating. Testes and ovaries distinguishable.

52

53 External genitalia still in sexless state but have begun to differentiate.

54 genital tubercle — urethral groove — anus ♀ or ♂

55 Growth & elaboration of structures occurring.

56 CR: 40 mm

57 Amniotic & chorionic sacs nearly obliterate uterine cavity.

58

59 Genitalia show some ♀ characteristics but still easily confused with ♂.

60 phallus — labium minus fold — labium majus fold — perineum ♀

61 Genitalia show fusion of urethral folds. Urethral groove extends into phallus.

62 phallus — urethral fold — scrotal fold — perineum ♂

63 CR: 50 mm

64 Face has human profile. Note growth of chin compared to day 44.

65

66 Face has human appearance.

67 clitoris — labium minus — urogenital groove — labium majus ♀

68 Genitalia have ♀ or ♂ characteristics but still not fully formed.

69 glans penis — urethral groove — scrotum ♂

70 CR: 61 mm

7

8

9

10

Figure 1–1. *Continued.*

4

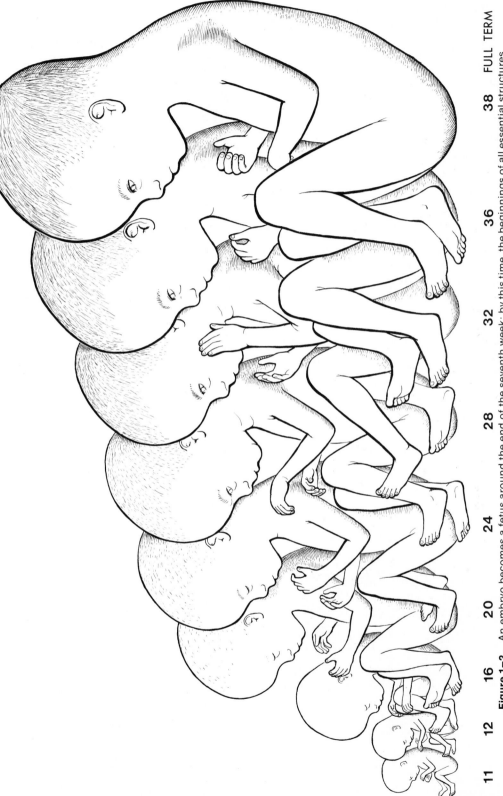

Figure 1-2. An embryo becomes a fetus around the end of the seventh week; by this time, the beginnings of all essential structures are present. The fetal period is characterized by growth and elaboration of structures. Sex is distinguishable externally at about 12 weeks. The 11- to 38-week fetuses are about half their actual size.

11   12   16   20   24   28   32   36   38   FULL TERM

especially in the pediatric age group, has made knowledge of human development more clinically significant. The understanding of most congenital malformations (e. g., cleft palate and cardiac defects) depends upon knowledge of normal development and the deviations that have occurred.

HISTORICAL HIGHLIGHTS

If I have seen further, it is by standing on the shoulders of giants.

Sir Isaac Newton[2]

This statement emphasizes that each new study of a problem rests on a base of knowledge established by earlier investigators. Every age gives explanations according to its knowledge and experience, and so we should be grateful for their ideas and neither sneer at them nor consider them as final. Man has always been interested in knowing how he originated, how he was born, and why some people develop abnormally.

The Greeks made important contributions to the science of embryology. The first recorded embryological studies are in the

---

[2]English mathematician, 1643–1727.

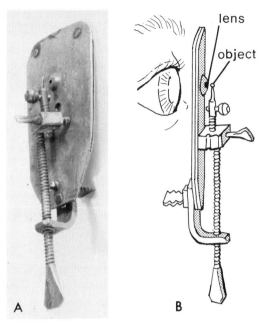

Figure 1–4. *A*, Photograph of a *1673 Leeuwenhoek microscope. B*, Drawing of a lateral view illustrating its use. The object was held in front of the lens on the point of the short rod, and the screw arrangement was used to adjust the object under the lens.

book of Hippocrates, the famous Greek physician of the fifth century B.C. In the fourth century B.C., Aristotle wrote the first known account of embryology, in which he described development of the chick and other embryos. Galen (second century A.D.) wrote a book entitled *On the Formation of the Foetus* in which he described the development and nutrition of fetuses.

Growth of science was slow during the Middle Ages, and no high points of embryological investigation are known to us. During the fifteenth century, Leonardo da Vinci made accurate drawings of dissections of the pregnant uterus and associated fetal membranes (Fig. 1–3).

In 1651 Harvey studied chick embryos with simple lenses and made observations on the circulation of blood. Early microscopes were simple (Fig. 1–4), but they opened a new field of observation. In 1672 de Graaf observed little chambers[3] in the rabbit's uterus and concluded that they came from organs he called ovaries.

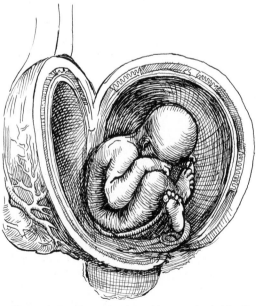

Figure 1–3. Reproduction of Leonardo da Vinci's drawing showing a fetus in an opened uterus.

---

[3]Undoubtedly what we now call blastocysts.

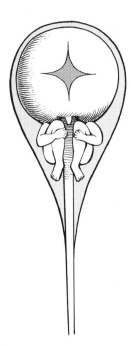

Figure 1–5. Copy of a seventeenth century drawing by Hartsoeker of a sperm. The miniature human being within it was thought to enlarge after it entered an ovum.

Malpighi, in 1675, studying what he believed to be unfertilized hen's eggs, observed early embryos. As a result, he thought the egg contained a miniature chick. In 1677 Hamm and Leeuwenhoek, using an improved microscope, first observed human sperms, but they did not understand the sperm's role in fertilization: they thought it contained a miniature human being (Fig. 1–5). Around 1775, Spallanzani showed that both the ovum and the sperm were necessary for initiation of a new individual. From his experiments, he concluded that the sperm was the fertilizing agent.

Great advances were made in embryology when the cell theory was established in 1839 by Schleiden and Schwann. The concept that the body was composed of cells and cell products soon led to the realization that the embryo developed from a single cell, the zygote.

Flemming observed chromosomes in 1878 and suggested their probable role in fertilization. In 1883 von Beneden observed that mature germ cells have a reduced number of chromosomes. The first signifi-cant observations on human chromosomes were made by von Winiwarter in 1912. In 1923 Painter concluded that there were 48 chromosomes. This number was universally accepted until 1956, when Tjio and Levan reported finding only 46 chromosomes. This number is now universally accepted.

DESCRIPTIVE TERMS

In descriptive anatomy and embryology, several terms of position and direction are used, and various planes of the body are referred to in sections. All descriptions of the adult are based on the assumption that the body is erect, with the arms by the sides and the palms directed forward (Fig. 1–6*A*). This is called the *anatomical position*. The terms *anterior* or *ventral* and *posterior* or *dorsal* are used to describe the front or back of the body or limbs, and the relations of structures within the body to one another. In embryos, dorsal and ventral are nearly always used (Fig. 1–6*B*).

Superior or *cranial* and *inferior* or *caudal* are used to indicate the relative levels of different structures. In embryos, cranial and caudal are commonly used to denote relationships to the head and tail ends, respectively. The term *rostral* is used to indicate the relationships of structures to the nose (Fig. 1–6*E*). Distances from the source of attachment of a structure are designated as *proximal* or *distal;* e.g., in the lower limb the knee is proximal to the ankle and the ankle is distal to the knee.

The *median plane* is a vertical plane passing through the center of the body, dividing it into right and left halves (Fig. 1–6*C*). The terms *lateral* and *medial* refer to structures which are respectively further from or nearer to the median plane of the body. A *sagittal plane* is any vertical plane passing through the body parallel to the median plane (Fig. 1–6*C*). A *transverse (horizontal) plane* refers to any plane that is at right angles to both the median and frontal planes (Fig. 1–6*D*). A *frontal (coronal) plane* is any vertical plane that intersects the median plane at a right angle; it divides the body into front (anterior or ventral) and back (posterior or dorsal) parts (Fig. 1–6*E*).

Various terms are used to describe sections of embryos made through the aforementioned planes. A *median (midsagittal) sec-*

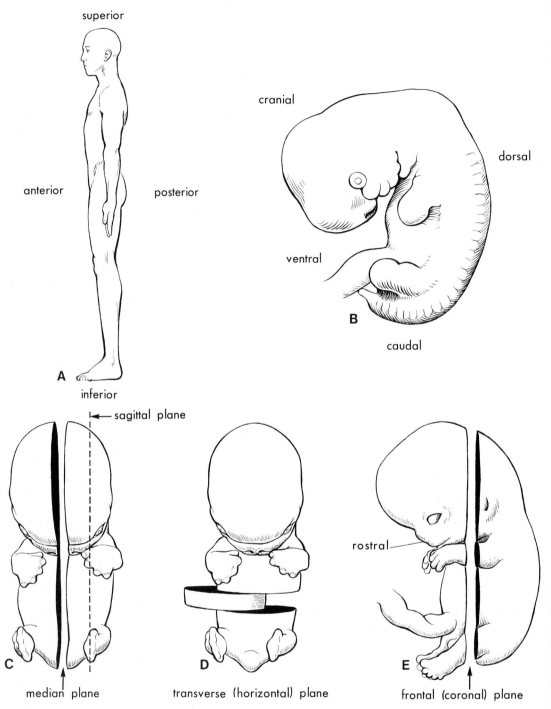

Figure 1–6. Drawings illustrating descriptive terms of position, direction and planes of the body. *A,* Lateral view of a human adult in the anatomical position. *B,* Lateral view of a five-week embryo. *C and D,* Ventral views of six-week embryos. *E,* Lateral view of a seven-week embryo.

tion is one cut through the median plane. Longitudinal sections parallel to the median plane, but not through it, are called sagittal sections. A vertical section through the frontal (coronal) plane is known as a *frontal (coronal) section.* Sections through the transverse plane are called *transverse (horizontal) sections,* or simply *cross sections. Oblique sections* are neither perpendicular nor horizontal, but are slanted or inclined.

2

REPRODUCTION

Bisexual reproduction is characteristic of all vertebrate species. Human reproduction, like that of most animals, involves the fusion of sex cells or gametes—an ovum or egg from the female and a sperm from the male. The reproductive system in both sexes is designed to insure the successful union of the sperm and the ovum.

THE REPRODUCTIVE ORGANS

The Female Reproductive Organs

The ova are produced by two oval-shaped *ovaries* located in the upper part of the pelvic cavity, one on each side of the uterus (Fig. 2–1*A*). When released from the ovary at *ovulation* (see Fig. 2–8), the ovum passes into one of two trumpet-shaped *uterine tubes* (Figs. 2–1*A* and 2–2*A*). These tubes open into the upper corners of the pear-shaped uterus (or womb), which contains and nourishes the developing child until birth.

Structure of the Uterus (Fig. 2–2). The uterine wall consists of three layers: (1) a very thin outer layer or *perimetrium;* (2) a thick, smooth-muscle layer or *myometrium;* and (3) a thin, inner lining layer or *endometrium.* Three layers of the endometrium can be distinguished microscopically: (1) a thin, superficial *compact layer* of densely packed, swollen connective tissue around the necks of the glands: (2) a thick *spongy layer* of fluid-filled or edematous connective tissue containing the dilated, tortuous bodies of the glands; and (3) a thin *basal layer* containing the blind ends of the glands. The compact and spongy layers disintegrate and are shed at *menstruation* and after a birth, and so are commonly called the *functional layer.*

The vagina is a muscular tube that passes to the exterior from the lower end of the uterus, called the *cervix.* The vagina is the basic female organ in sexual intercourse in that it receives the male organ or penis (see Fig. 2–9). It also serves as a temporary receptacle for the sperms before they begin their passage through the uterus and uterine tubes.

The External Sex Organs. These are known collectively as the *vulva* (Fig. 2–3). Two external folds of skin, the *labia majora* (larger lips), enclose the opening of the vagina. Inside these folds are two smaller lips called *labia minora.* The *clitoris* is at the junction of these folds; it is a small, erectile organ that is homologous to the penis.

The Male Reproductive Organs

The sperms are produced in the *testes,* two oval-shaped glands located in the *scrotum,* a loose pouch of skin (Fig. 2–1*B*). Each testis consists of many highly coiled *seminiferous tubules* which produce the sperms. The sperms pass into a single, complexly coiled tube, the *epididymis,* where they are stored. From the lower end of each epididymis, a long straight tube, the *ductus deferens* (vas deferens), passes from the scrotum through the inguinal canal into the abdominal cavity. It then descends into the pelvis where it fuses with the duct of the *seminal vesicle* to form the *ejaculatory duct* which enters the *urethra.* The urethra is a tube leading from the urinary bladder to the outside of the body; its terminal part runs through the

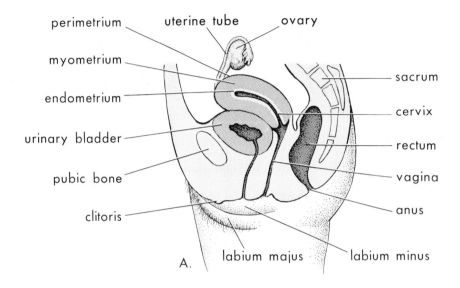

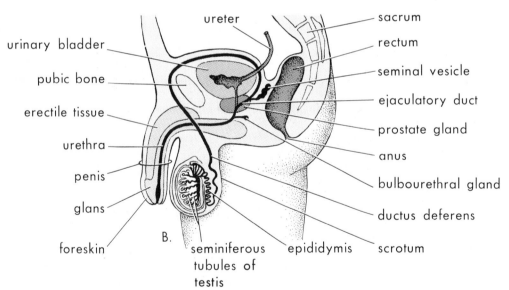

Figure 2–1. Schematic sagittal sections of the pelvic region showing the reproductive organs. *A*, Female. *B*, Male.

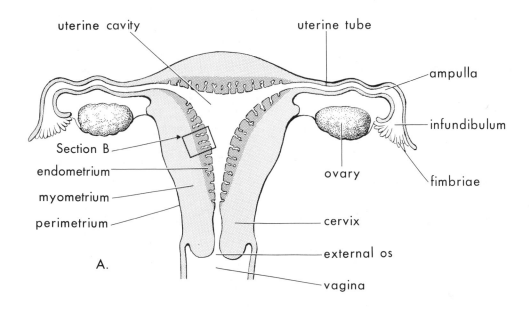

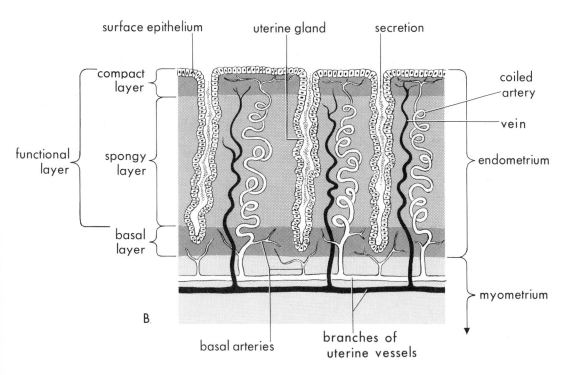

Figure 2-2. *A*, Diagrammatic frontal section of the uterus and uterine tubes. The ovaries and vagina are also indicated. *B*, Detail of the area outlined in *A*.

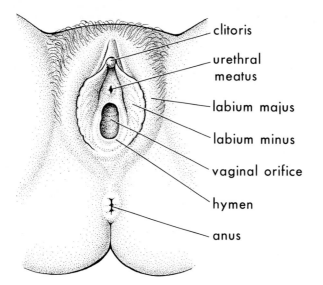

clitoris

urethral meatus

labium majus

labium minus

vaginal orifice

hymen

anus

Figure 2–3. The external female genital organs, known collectively as the vulva. The opening at the lower end of the alimentary canal, the anus, is also shown.

penis, the external reproductive organ. Within the penis the urethra is flanked by three columns of spongy erectile tissue. During sexual excitement this tissue becomes filled with blood under increased pressure; this causes the penis to become erect and thus able to enter the vagina. Ejaculation of *semen* (sperms in seminal fluid produced by various glands, e.g., the seminal vesicles and prostate) occurs when the penis is further stimulated.

THE GERM CELLS OR GAMETES

The *sperm* and the *ovum* (the male and female germ cells or gametes) are highly specialized *sex cells* (Fig. 2–4 and 2–5). They contain half the usual number of chromosomes. The number of chromosomes is reduced by the process of *meiosis* which occurs during the formation of gametes or *gametogenesis*, a process known as spermatogenesis in males and *oogenesis* in females (Fig. 2–5). Meiosis consists of two cell divisions during which the chromosome number is reduced to half that present in other cells in the body. During the final stages of maturation, the two chromosomes in each of the 23 pairs are separated from each other and distributed to different cells. Therefore each mature germ cell (sperm or ovum) contains one member of each pair of the chromo-

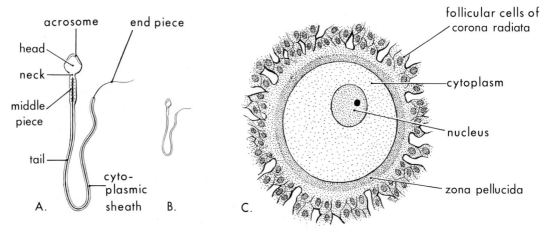

acrosome

end piece

head

neck

middle piece

tail

cyto-plasmic sheath

A.

B.

C.

follicular cells of corona radiata

cytoplasm

nucleus

zona pellucida

Figure 2–4. *A,* Drawing showing the main parts of a human sperm (×1250). The head, composed mostly of the nucleus, is covered by the acrosome. *B,* A sperm drawn to about the same scale as the ovum. *C,* Drawing of a human ovum (×200), surrounded by the zona pellucida and corona radiata.

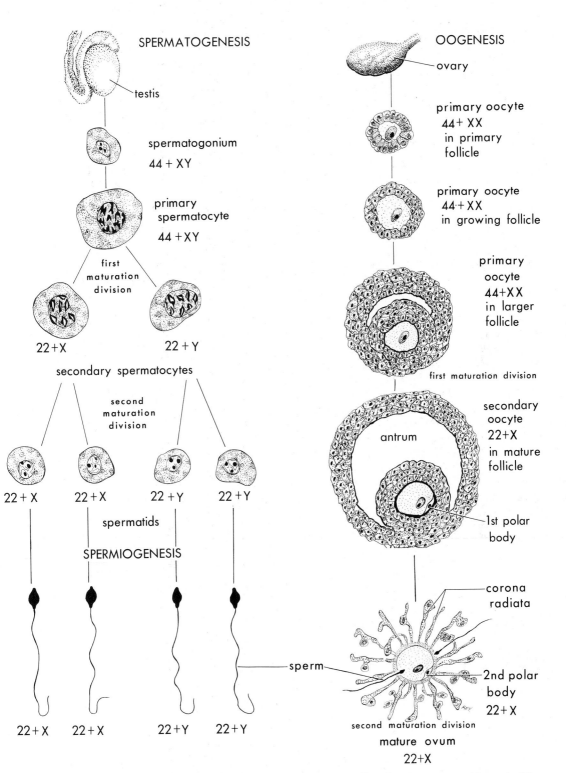

SPERMATOGENESIS

testis

spermatogonium
44 + XY

primary
spermatocyte
44 + XY

first
maturation
division

22 + X   22 + Y

secondary spermatocytes

second
maturation
division

22 + X   22 + X   22 + Y   22 + Y

spermatids

SPERMIOGENESIS

22 + X   22 + X   22 + Y   22 + Y

OOGENESIS

ovary

primary oocyte
44 + XX
in primary
follicle

primary oocyte
44 + XX
in growing follicle

primary
oocyte
44 + XX
in larger
follicle

first maturation division

secondary
oocyte
22 + X
in mature
follicle

antrum

1st polar
body

corona
radiata

sperm

2nd polar
body
22 + X

second maturation division

mature ovum
22 + X

Figure 2–5. Drawings comparing spermatogenesis and oogenesis. The chromosome complement of the germ cells is indicated at each stage. Note that (1) following the two maturation divisions, the diploid number of chromosomes, 46, is reduced to the haploid number, 23; and (2) *four sperms* form from one primary spermatocyte, whereas only *one ovum* results from maturation of a primary oocyte.

somes present in the immature germ cell (primary spermatocyte or primary oocyte).

Spermatogenesis (Sperm Development)

The early germ cells, or *spermatogonia*, which have been dormant in the seminiferous tubules of the testes since the fetal period, begin to increase in number at *puberty*. After several mitotic or ordinary cell divisions, the spermatogonia grow and undergo gradual changes which transform them into *primary spermatocytes* (Fig. 2–5), the largest germ cells in the seminiferous tubules. Each primary spermatocyte subsequently undergoes a reduction division,[1] called the *first maturation division*, to form two haploid[2] *secondary spermatocytes* which are about half the size of primary spermatocytes. Subsequently, these secondary spermatocytes undergo a *second maturation division* to form four haploid *spermatids* which are about half the size of secondary spermatocytes. During this division, there is no further reduction in the number of chromosomes; although part of meiosis, it is like a mitotic division. The spermatids are gradually transformed into *mature sperms* by an extensive process of differentiation known as *spermiogenesis*. Spermatogenesis, including spermiogenesis, requires two to three weeks for completion and normally continues throughout the reproductive life of the male.

Oogenesis (Ovum Development)

During early fetal life, primitive ova or *oogonia* proliferate by mitotic division. These oogonia enlarge to form *primary oocytes* before birth (Fig. 2–5). As the primary oocyte forms, ovarian stromal cells surround it and form a single layer of flattened follicular cells. The primary oocyte enclosed by this layer of follicular cells constitutes a *primary follicle* (Fig. 2–6A).

---

[1]This process of reduction by an atypical method of cell division is called meiosis; it consists of two specialized divisions called the first and second maturation divisions.

[2]In man, body cells and early sex cells have 46 chromosomes (the diploid number). Mature sex cells have 23 chromosomes (the haploid number).

The primary oocytes remain dormant in the ovaries until puberty and then increase in size. A deeply staining membrane, the *zona pellucida*, forms around it (Figs. 2–4C and 2–6B and C). Shortly before ovulation the primary oocyte completes the *first maturation division*. Unlike the corresponding stage of spermatogenesis, however, the division of cytoplasm is unequal. The *secondary oocyte* receives almost all the cytoplasm (Fig. 2–6B) and the *first polar body* or cell receives hardly any (Fig. 2–5); this small nonfunctional cell subsequently degenerates. At ovulation the nucleus of the secondary oocyte begins the *second maturation division*, but progresses only to metaphase, where division is arrested. If *fertilization occurs*, the second maturation division is completed and most cytoplasm is again retained by one cell, the *mature ovum* (Fig. 2–5). The other cell, called the *second polar body*, is very small and soon degenerates.

The ovum released at ovulation is surrounded by the *zona pellucida* and a layer of follicular cells called the *corona radiata* (Fig. 2–4C). Compared with ordinary cells, it is truly large and is barely visible to the unaided eye as a tiny speck. At least two million primary oocytes are usually present in the ovaries of a newborn female infant. Many of these regress during childhood so that by puberty only 10,000 to 30,000 remain. Of these, only about 400 mature and are expelled at ovulation.

Comparison of the Sperm and Ovum

The sperm and ovum are dissimilar in several ways because of their adaptation to specialized roles. The ovum is massive compared to the sperm (Fig. 2–4) and is immotile, whereas the microscopic sperm is highly motile. The ovum has an abundance of cytoplasm containing yolk granules which provide nutrition during the first week of development. The sperm bears little resemblance to an ovum or to any other cell because of its sparse cytoplasm and specialization for motility.

With respect to sex chromosome constitution, there are two kinds of normal sperm (Fig. 2–5): 22 autosomes plus an X chromosome; and 22 autosomes plus a Y chromosome. However, there is only one kind of normal ovum: 22 autosomes plus an X chromosome.

follicular cells   nucleus of primary oocyte   zona pellucida   cumulus oophorus

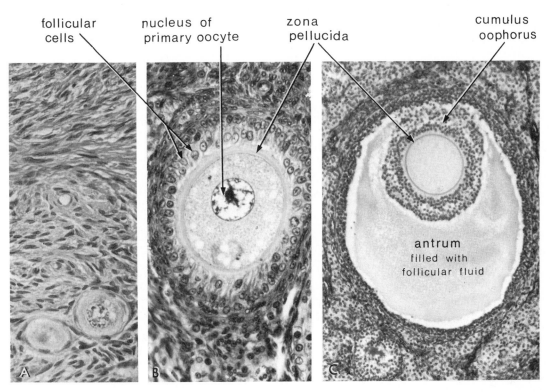

antrum
filled with
follicular fluid

Figure 2–6. Photomicrographs of sections from adult human ovaries. *A,* Ovarian cortex showing two primary follicles (×250). *B,* Growing follicle containing a primary oocyte, surrounded by the zona pellucida and a stratified layer of follicular cells (×250). *C,* An almost mature follicle with a large antrum. The oocyte, embedded in the cumulus oophorus, does not show a nucleus because it has been sectioned tangentially (×100). (From Leeson, T. S., and Leeson, C. R.: *Histology,* 2nd ed., 1970. Courtesy of the W. B. Saunders Co.) See color film loop SB/J/1, entitled "Growth of the oocyte and development of the ovarian follicle."

REPRODUCTIVE CYCLES

Commencing at puberty and normally continuing throughout the reproductive years, human females undergo monthly *reproductive* or *sexual cycles* involving the hypothalamus, pituitary gland, ovaries and uterus (Fig. 2–7). These cycles prepare the female reproductive system for pregnancy. Small blood vessels carry "releasing factors" from the hypothalamus to the anterior pituitary gland which regulate this gland's production of gonadotropins: *follicle-stimulating hormone* (FSH) and *luteinizing hormone* (LH).

The Ovarian Cycle

The gonadotropins produce cyclic changes in the ovaries (development of follicles, ovulation and corpus luteum formation) known as the *ovarian cycle.*

Follicular Development (Figs. 2–5 and 2–6). Development of a follicle is characterized by (1) growth and differentiation of the primary oocyte, (2) proliferation of follicular cells, and (3) development of a connective tissue capsule, the *theca folliculi.* The follicle soon becomes oval in shape and the ovum eccentric in position because the follicular cells proliferate more rapidly on one side. Subsequently, fluid-filled spaces appear around the follicular cells; these spaces soon coalesce to form a large fluid-filled cavity, the *antrum.* An eccentric mound, the *cumulus oophorus,* forms where the oocyte lies within the follicular cells.

Development of follicles is initially induced by FSH, but final stages of maturation require LH as well. Growing follicles produce *estrogen,* a female sex hormone which regulates development and function of the reproductive organs. Estrogen also appears to stimulate gonadotropin (LH) release by the pituitary.

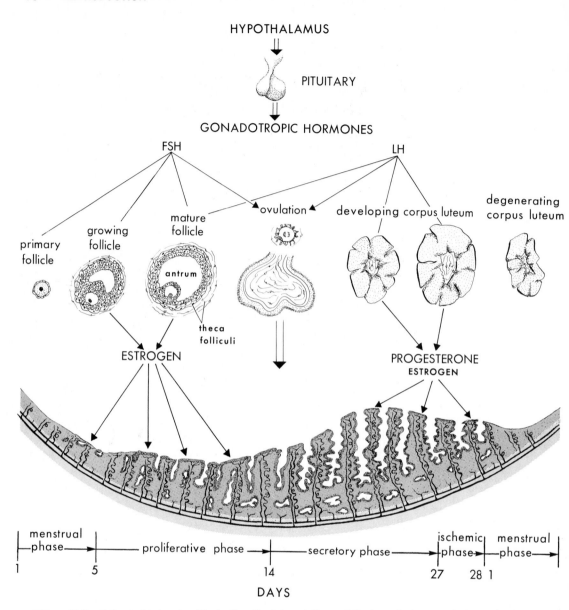

Figure 2–7. Schematic drawing illustrating the interrelations of the hypothalamus, pituitary gland, ovaries and endometrium. One complete menstrual cycle and the beginning of another are shown.

Ovulation (Fig. 2–8). Ovulation usually occurs about two weeks before the next expected menstrual period, i.e., about 14 days after the first day of the menstrual period in the typical 28-day cycle (Fig. 2–7). Under FSH and LH influence, the follicle undergoes a sudden growth spurt, producing a swelling on the surface of the ovary. A small oval avascular spot, the *stigma*, soon appears on this swelling. During ovulation the ovarian surface ruptures at the stigma and the oocyte is expelled with the follicular fluid from the follicle and the ovary. The released ovum or oocyte is surrounded by the *zona pellucida* and one or more layers of radially arranged follicular cells which form the *corona radiata* (Fig. 2–4C).

The Corpus Luteum. At ovulation the walls of the follicle collapse (Fig. 2–8D) and under LH influence, develop into a glandular structure known as the corpus luteum (Figs. 2–7 and 2–8D). It secretes *progesterone*

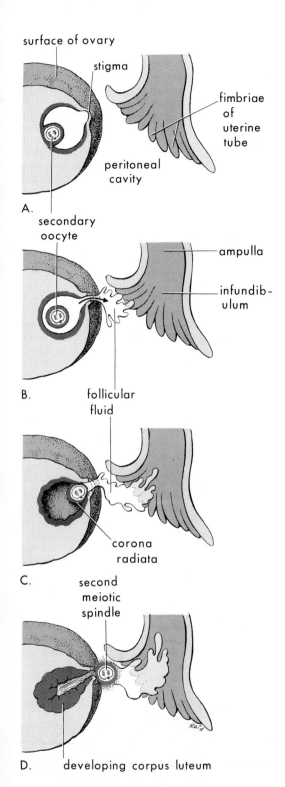

surface of ovary

stigma

fimbriae
of
uterine
tube

peritoneal
cavity

A.

secondary
oocyte

ampulla

infundib-
ulum

B. follicular
fluid

corona
radiata

C. second
meiotic
spindle

D. developing corpus luteum

Figure 2–8. Diagrams illustrating ovulation. The stigma ruptures and the oocyte is expelled with the follicular fluid. See color film loop SB/J/2S, entitled "Ovulation."

and some estrogen. These hormones, particularly progesterone, cause the endometrial glands to secrete and prepare the endometrium for implantation of the blastocyst (the developing embryo). If the ovum is fertilized, the corpus luteum enlarges to form a *corpus luteum of pregnancy* and increases its hormone production. If the ovum is not fertilized, the corpus luteum begins to degenerate about nine days after ovulation (Fig. 2–7) and is called a *corpus luteum of menstruation.*

The Menstrual Cycle

The periodic changes occurring in the endometrium constitute the uterine cycle, commonly referred to as the menstrual cycle because menstruation is an obvious event. The common length of a cycle is 28 days, but this may vary markedly from individual to individual and between cycles of the same individual.

Ovarian hormones cause cyclic changes in the structure of the reproductive tract, notably the endometrium. Although divided into four phases (Fig. 2–7), it must be stressed that the menstrual cycle is a *continuous* process; each phase gradually passing into the next one.

The Menstrual Phase. The first day of menstruation is counted as the beginning of the menstrual cycle. The functional layer of the uterine wall (Fig. 2–2*B*) is sloughed off and discarded during menstruation which typically occurs at 28-day intervals and lasts for three to five days.

The Proliferative Phase. Estrogen causes regeneration of the epithelium, lengthening of the glands, and multiplication of connective tissue cells.

The Secretory Phase. Progesterone induces the glands to become tortuous and to secrete profusely, and the connective tissue to become grossly edematous (a condition in which there are large amounts of fluid in the intercellular spaces).

The Ischemic Phase.[3] Extensive vascular changes occur about 13 to 14 days after ovulation. The coiled arteries constrict in-

[3]If pregnancy occurs, this phase does not take place. The secretory phase gradually passes into a *pregnancy phase.* After termination of pregnancy, the menstrual cycles resume after a variable period.

termittently, the functional layer becomes pale, and the endometrium shrinks as a result of anemia and anoxia. Bleeding soon occurs and the menstrual phase begins again.

GERM CELL TRANSPORT

Ovum Transport. The ovum leaves the ovary with the escaping follicular fluid. The finger-like *fimbriae* of the uterine tube (Fig. 2–8*A*) move to and fro over the ovary and "sweep" the ovum into the tube. The ovum passes into the *ampulla* of the tube (Fig. 2–8*B*), largely as a result of the beating action of cilia on some tubal epithelial cells, but partly by muscular contractions of the tubal wall.

Sperm Transport. About 300 to 500 million of the sperms stored in the epididymis are deposited in the vagina during the process of ejaculation occurring during sexual intercourse (Fig. 2–9). The sperms pass by movements of their tails into the cervical canal, but passage of the sperms through the remainder of the uterus and the uterine tubes results mainly from contractions of the walls of these organs. It is not known how long it takes sperms to reach the fertilization site, but the time of transport is probably not more than an hour. Only a few hundred sperms reach the fertilization site in each uterine tube.

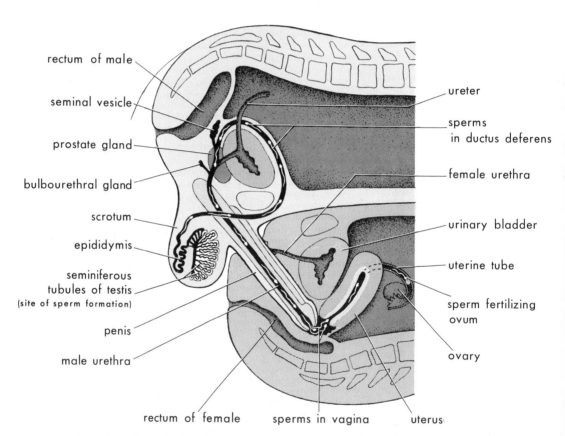

Figure 2–9. Schematic sagittal section of the male and female pelvis showing the penis in the vagina. The sperms are produced in the seminiferous tubules of the testis and stored in the epididymis. During ejaculation the sperms pass along the ductus deferens and into the urethra where they mix with secretions from the seminal vesicles, prostate and bulbourethral glands. This mixture, called semen, is deposited in the upper portion of the vagina, close to the external opening of the uterus. The sperms pass through the cavity of the uterus and out to the outer third of the uterine tubes where fertilization occurs.

SUMMARY

Human reproduction involves the fusion of an ovum from a female and a sperm from a male. The reproductive system in both sexes is designed to insure the union of these sex (germ) cells. The ovum produced by the ovary is expelled from it at ovulation and passes into the uterine tube. The sperms are produced by the seminiferous tubules of the testes and stored in the epididymis. During the process of ejaculation, occurring during sexual intercourse, the sperms are deposited in the vagina. They soon pass through the cervical canal, the uterine cavity and along the uterine tube to the ampulla where fertilization occurs if an ovum is present.

3

THE FIRST WEEK OF DEVELOPMENT

Life begins for each of us at an unfelt, unknown, unhonored instant when a minute, wriggling sperm plunges into a mature egg.

M. S. Gilbert, 1963

Development begins at fertilization when a sperm fuses with an ovum or egg to form a *zygote*[1]; the first cell of a new human being. The zygote undergoes cell division and many complex changes occur before the developing human is able to live independently.

The ovum released at ovulation retains the capacity to be fertilized for up to 12 hours. Sperms in the female genital tract retain their ability to fertilize ova for up to 48 hours. Therefore, the *fertile period* during a woman's menstrual cycle is about 60 hours. This period varies in individual women, but generally the most fertile time is about the fourteenth day after the onset of menstruation in the usual 28-day cycle.

FERTILIZATION

Fertilization usually occurs in the intermediate dilated portion of the uterine tube called the *ampulla* (see Fig. 2–2A) and consists of the fusion of a sperm with an ovum (Fig. 3–1 and 3–2). Before this process can occur, a sperm must undergo a physiological change or "conditioning" called *capacitation* and a structural change known as the *acrosome reaction*. Capacitation may result

[1]From the Greek word *zygotos*, meaning "yoked together."

from the removal of a protective coating. During the acrosome reaction small perforations occur in the wall of the acrosome, a cap-like structure which covers the anterior half of the head of the sperm (Fig. 3–1B). These openings permit the escape of enzymes which digest a path for the sperm through the corona radiata and zona pellucida around the ovum.

Fertilization may be summarized as follows:

1. The sperm passes through the corona radiata (the cells surrounding the ovum).

2. The sperm penetrates the zona pellucida, digesting a path by the action of enzymes released from its acrosome.

3. The sperm head attaches to the surface of the ovum.

4. The ovum reacts to sperm contact in two ways: (a) the zona pellucida and the ovum's cell membrane change so that the entry of more sperms is prevented, and (b) the secondary oocyte completes the second meiotic division and expels the second polar body (Fig. 3–2B). The ovum is now mature and its nucleus is called the female pronucleus.

5. The sperm head enlarges to form the male pronucleus. The tail of the sperm degenerates (Fig. 3–2C).

6. The male and female pronuclei fuse in the center of the ovum where they come into contact, lose their nuclear membranes and their chromosomes intermingle (Fig. 3–2D).

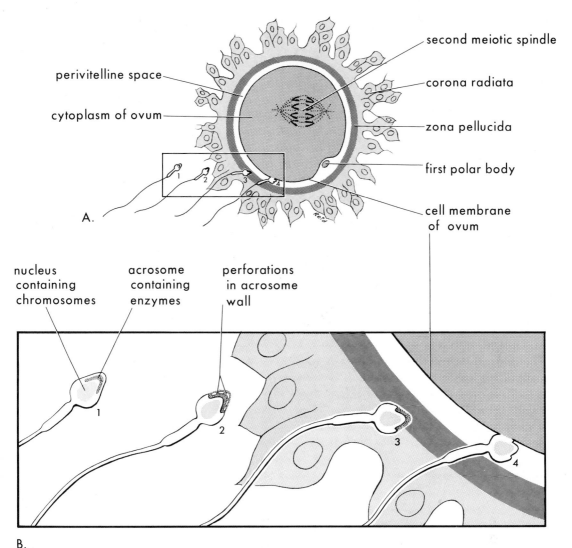

perivitelline space

cytoplasm of ovum

second meiotic spindle

corona radiata

zona pellucida

first polar body

cell membrane of ovum

A.

nucleus containing chromosomes

acrosome containing enzymes

perforations in acrosome wall

B.

Figure 3-1. Diagrams illustrating fertilization. The acrosome reaction and the penetration of a sperm into an ovum are shown. The detail of the area outlined in *A* is given in *B*: (1) sperm during capacitation, (2) sperm undergoing the acrosome reaction, (3) sperm digesting a path for itself by the action of enzymes released from the acrosome, (4) sperm head fusing with ovum.

Results of Fertilization

Restoration of the Diploid Number of Chromosomes. Fusion of the two germ cells (each with 23 chromosomes) produces a zygote, which is a diploid cell with 46 chromosomes, the normal number for the human species. One member of each of the 23 pairs of chromosomes is derived from each parent.

Species Variation. Because half the chromosomes come from the mother and the other half from the father, the zygote contains a new combination of chromosomes. Within each chromosome are numerous hereditary factors called *genes*, each of which differs from others and controls the inheritance of one or more characteristics. Consequently, fertilization forms the basis of biparental inheritance and insures variation of the human species.

Sex Determination. The embryo's sex is determined at fertilization by the kind of sperm that fertilizes the ovum. Fertilization

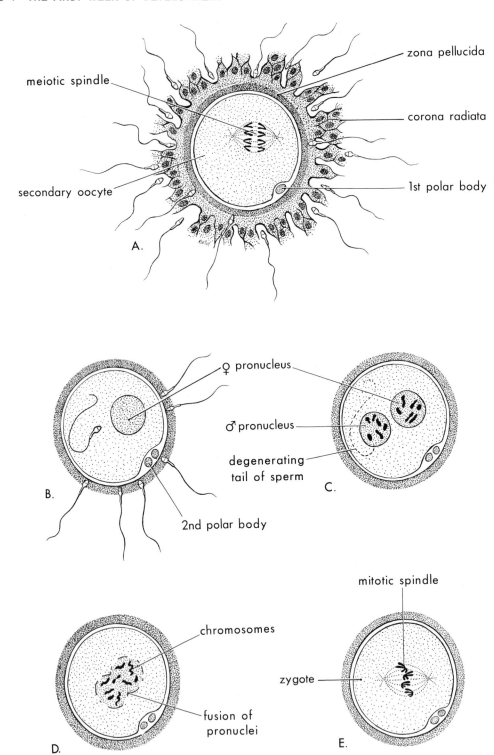

Figure 3–2. Diagrams illustrating fertilization. *A*, Secondary oocyte about to be fertilized. (Only four of the 23 chromosome pairs are shown.) *B*, The corona radiata has disappeared; a sperm has entered the ovum, and the second maturation division has occurred. *C*, The sperm head has enlarged to form the male pronucleus. *D*, The pronuclei are fusing. *E*, The chromosomes of the zygote are arranged on a mitotic spindle in preparation for the first cleavage division. See color film loop SB/J/3, entitled "Fertilization."

by an X-bearing sperm produces an XX zygote, which normally develops into a female, whereas fertilization by a Y-bearing sperm produces an XY zygote, which normally develops into a male. Sex determination is discussed further in Chapter 14.

Initiation of Cleavage. Fertilization of the ovum by a sperm also initiates early human development by stimulating the zygote to undergo division or cleavage into two blastomeres.

CLEAVAGE

As the zygote passes down the uterine tube, it undergoes cell division. Division of the zygote into two daughter cells, called *blastomeres* (Fig. 3–3A), begins shortly after

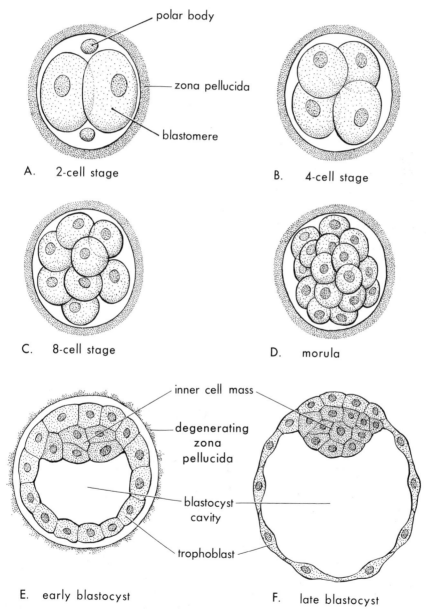

A. 2-cell stage

B. 4-cell stage

C. 8-cell stage

D. morula

E. early blastocyst

F. late blastocyst

Figure 3–3. Drawings illustrating cleavage of the zygote and formation of the blastocyst. *E* and *F* are sections of blastocysts. Note that the zona pellucida has disappeared by the last blastocyst stage (about five days). See color film loop SB/J/4, entitled "Cleavage and the formation of the blastocyst."

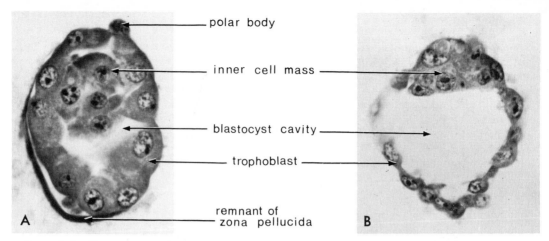

Figure 3–4. Photomicrographs of sections of human blastocysts recovered from the uterine cavity (×600). *A*, Four days; the blastocyst cavity is just beginning to form and the zona pellucida is deficient over part of the blastocyst. *B*, Four and a half days; the blastocyst cavity has enlarged and the inner cell mass and trophoblast are clearly defined. The zona pellucida has disappeared. (From Hertig, A. T., Rock, J., and Adams, E. C.: *Amer. J. Anat. 98*:435, 1956. Courtesy of Carnegie Institution of Washington.)

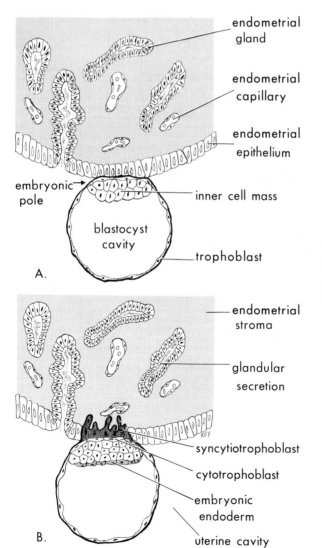

Figure 3–5. Drawings of sections illustrating early stages of implantation. *A*, Six days; the trophoblast is attached to the endometrial epithelium at the embryonic pole of the blastocyst. *B*, Seven days; the syncytiotrophoblast has penetrated the endometrial epithelium.

fertilization. Subsequent divisions follow rapidly upon one another, forming progressively smaller blastomeres (Fig. 3–3*B* to *D*). The term cleavage is used to describe the process of rapid mitotic divisions. By about three days, a solid ball of 16 or so blastomeres has formed, which is called a *morula*.[2] It enters the uterus and fluid passes into the morula from the uterine cavity and collects between its cells. As the fluid increases, it separates these cells into two parts: (1) an outer cell mass called the *trophoblast*[3] and (2) a group of centrally located cells known as the *inner cell mass* (or embryoblast[4]).

By the fourth day the fluid-filled spaces fuse to form a single large space known as the *blastocyst cavity*. This converts the morula into a *blastocyst* (Figs. 3–3*E* and 3–4). The inner cell mass (future embryo) projects into

the blastocyst cavity and the trophoblast forms the wall of the blastocyst (Fig. 3–3*F*). The blastocyst lies free in the uterine secretions for about two days. On about the fifth day the *zona pellucida* degenerates and disappears (Fig. 3–3*E* and *F*). The blastocyst attaches to the maternal uterine epithelium on about the sixth day (Fig. 3–5*A*). The trophoblastic cells soon begin to destroy the adjacent endometrial cells (Fig. 3–5*B*).

As invasion of the trophoblast proceeds, two cell layers form: (1) an inner *cytotrophoblast* (cellular trophoblast), and (2) an outer *syncytiotrophoblast* (syncytial trophoblast). The finger-like processes of the syncytiotrophoblast penetrate the endometrial epithelium and invade the endometrial stroma. By the end of the first week, the blastocyst is superficially implanted in the lining (endometrium) of the uterus (Fig. 3–5*B*).

As the blastocyst implants, early differentiation of the embryo (inner cell mass) occurs. A layer of cells, called the *embryonic endoderm*, appears on the free surface of the inner cell mass (Fig. 3–5*B*). The endoderm later gives rise to the epithelium of the primitive gut (see Fig. 6–2 and Chapter 13).

---

[2]From Latin *morus*, meaning "mulberry." The morula is a mulberry-like cellular mass.

[3]From Greek *trophe*, meaning "nutrition" and *blastos*, meaning "germ" or "bud"; the trophoblast later forms the major part of the placenta.

[4]The inner cell mass gives rise to the embryo.

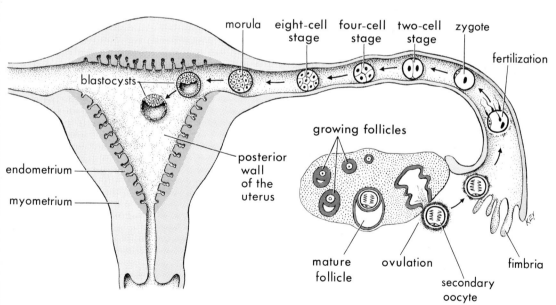

Figure 3–6. Diagrammatic summary of the ovarian cycle, fertilization and development during the first week. The numbers indicate days after fertilization. The ovum is released from the ovary at ovulation and passes into the uterine tube where it is met and fertilized by a sperm. The zygote divides repeatedly as it passes down the uterine tube and becomes a morula. The morula enters the uterus, develops a cavity and becomes a blastocyst. The blastocyst begins to invade the endometrial lining of the uterus.

SUMMARY

Fertilization usually occurs in the ampulla of the uterine tube. The process is complete when the haploid male and female pronuclei fuse to form the diploid *zygote* (Fig. 3–6). This cell is the beginning of a new human being. As it passes down the uterine tube, the zygote undergoes cell division or *cleavage* into a number of smaller cells called *blastomeres*. About three days after fertilization, a ball of 16 or so blastomeres, the *morula*, enters the uterus. A cavity soon forms in the morula, converting it into a *blastocyst*. The zona pellucida disappears and the blastocyst contacts the lining of the uterus. The trophoblastic cells invade the uterine epithelium and underlying endometrial stroma. By the end of the first week, the blastocyst is superficially implanted in the endometrial lining of the uterus.

4

THE SECOND
WEEK OF
DEVELOPMENT

Implantation or embedding of the blastocyst in the endometrial lining of the uterus is completed during the second week of development. Changes occur in the inner cell mass which result in the formation of a thick plate called the *embryonic disc;* this disc will differentiate into the embryo. The *amniotic cavity, yolk sac, connecting stalk* and *chorion* also begin to develop during the second week.

The actively erosive *trophoblast* continues to invade the endometrium containing capillaries and glands, and the blastocyst slowly sinks within the endometrial lining of the uterus. As more trophoblast contacts the endometrium, the trophoblast proliferates and differentiates into two layers (Fig. 4–1*A*). The *cytotrophoblast* is composed of cells, whereas the *syncytiotrophoblast* is a thick multinucleated protoplasmic mass. Isolated spaces, or *lacunae*, appear in the syncytiotrophoblast which soon become filled with blood from ruptured maternal capillaries and secretions from eroded endometrial glands (Fig. 4–1*C*). This nutritive fluid or *embryotroph* passes to the early embryo by diffusion.

Small spaces appear between the inner cell mass and the invading trophoblast. These spaces soon coalesce to form a slit-like *amniotic cavity* (Fig. 4–1*A*).

FORMATION OF THE BILAMINAR EMBRYO

As the amniotic cavity forms, changes occur in the inner cell mass, resulting in the formation of a flattened, essentially circular *embryonic disc*. It consists of two layers: *embryonic ectoderm* related to the amniotic cavity, and *embryonic endoderm* related to the blastocyst cavity. As the amniotic cavity enlarges, a thin epithelial roof, the *amnion*, forms from cytotrophoblastic cells. The embryonic ectoderm forms the floor of the amniotic cavity and is continuous peripherally with the amnion (Fig. 4–1*C*). Concurrently, other cells from the trophoblast form a thin *exocoelomic (Heuser's) membrane* which encloses a cavity known as the primitive *yolk sac* (Fig. 4–1*C*). The human yolk sac contains no yolk, but it is an essential structure that has an important role during later development of the embryo (see Chapter 8). Some trophoblastic cells give rise to a layer of loosely arranged tissue around the amnion and the primitive yolk sac. This is called *extraembryonic mesoderm.*

The *10-day conceptus* (the embryo and its membranes) lies completely within the endometrial lining of the uterus (Fig. 4–2). For a day or so a defect may be recognized by a *closing plug* consisting of a blood clot and

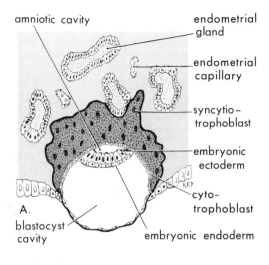

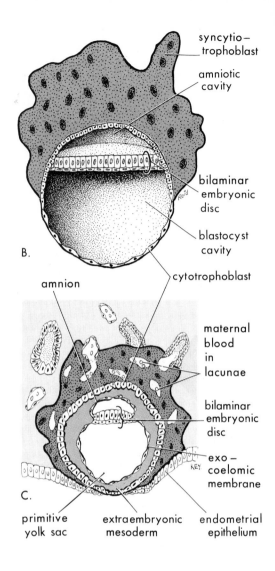

Figure 4–1. *A,* Drawing of a section through an eight-day blastocyst partially implanted in the endometrium. *B,* An enlarged three-dimensional sketch of this blastocyst after removal from the endometrium. Note the extensive syncytiotrophoblast at the embryonic pole. *C,* Drawing of a section through a blastocyst of about nine days implanted in the endometrium. (Based on Hertig and Rock, 1945.)

cellular debris. By day 11 isolated spaces are visible within the extraembryonic mesoderm; these spaces rapidly fuse to form large isolated cavities of *extraembryonic coelom* (Figs. 4–2*B* and 4–4*B*). By day 12 the epithelium covers over the blastocyst, producing a minute elevation or wart-like bulge on the endometrial surface (Fig. 4–3).

Meanwhile adjacent trophoblastic lacunae have fused to form intercommunicating *lacunar networks* (Fig. 4–2*B*), the primitive *intervillous spaces* of the placenta (see Chapter 8). The endometrial capillaries around the implanted embryo have also become dilated to form *sinusoids* and some have been eroded by the trophoblast. Maternal blood then seeps into the lacunar networks and soon begins to flow slowly through the lacunar system, establishing a primitive *uteroplacental circulation.*

By the end of the second week, a defect is no longer present in the endometrial epithelium (Fig. 4–5*A*). *Primary villi* (finger-like projections) of the chorion have also formed (Fig. 4–6). These will later differentiate into the chorionic villi of the placenta (see Chapter 8). The isolated coelomic spaces in the extraembryonic mesoderm have now fused to form a single large extraembryonic coelom. This fluid-filled cavity surrounds the amnion and yolk sac, except where the amnion is attached to the trophoblast by the *connecting (body) stalk* (Fig. 4–5*B*). As the extraembryonic coelom forms, the primitive yolk sac decreases in size, resulting in a smaller *secondary yolk sac.*

(Text continued on page 32.)

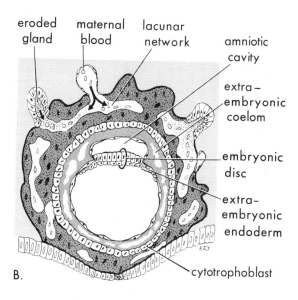

Figure 4–2. Drawings of sections through completely implanted blastocysts. *A*, 10 days. *B*, 12 days. Note that some endometrial sinusoids and glands are in open communication with the lacunar networks. As the trophoblast erodes the capillaries and glands, both blood and glandular secretions soon fill the lacunae and lacunar networks in the trophoblast. This mixture, called embryotroph, provides a source of nutrient for the developing embryo. (Based on Hertig and Rock, 1941.)

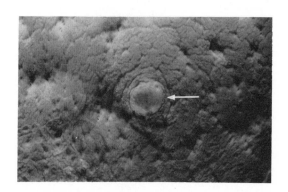

Figure 4–3. Photograph of the endometrial surface showing the implantation site of a human embryo of about 12 days; the implanted conceptus causes a small elevation (arrow) (×8). (From Hertig, A. T., and Rock, J.: *Contr. Embryol. Carneg. Instn., Wash. 29*:127, 1941. Courtesy of the Carnegie Institution of Washington.)

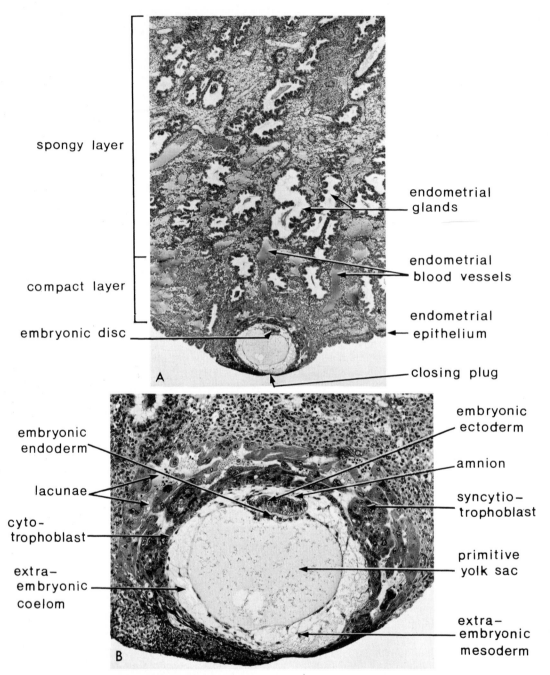

spongy layer

compact layer

embryonic disc

endometrial glands

endometrial blood vessels

endometrial epithelium

closing plug

embryonic endoderm

lacunae

cyto-trophoblast

extra-embryonic coelom

embryonic ectoderm

amnion

syncytio-trophoblast

primitive yolk sac

extra-embryonic mesoderm

Figure 4–4. *A,* A section through the implantation site of the 12-day embryo shown in Figure 4–3. The embryo is embedded in the compact layer of the endometrium (×30). *B,* Higher magnification of the conceptus and surrounding endometrium (×100). (From Hertig, A. T., and Rock, J.: *Contr. Embryol. Carneg. Instn., Wash.* 29:127, 1941. Courtesy of the Carnegie Institution of Washington.)

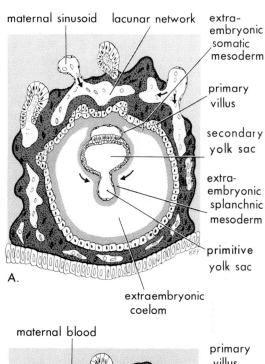

maternal sinusoid   lacunar network   extra-embryonic somatic mesoderm

primary villus

secondary yolk sac

extra-embryonic splanchnic mesoderm

primitive yolk sac

A.

extraembryonic coelom

Figure 4–5. Drawings of sections through implanted human embryos, based mainly on Hertig *et al.,* 1956. *A,* 13 days, illustrating the decrease in relative size of the primitive yolk sac and the early appearance of primary villi at the embryonic pole. Note the maternal blood in the lacunar networks. *B,* 14 days, showing the secondary yolk sac and the location of the endodermal prochordal plate. The prochordal plate indicates the site of the future mouth. *C,* Detail of the prochordal plate area outlined in *B.* See color film loop SB/J/5S, entitled "Implantation."

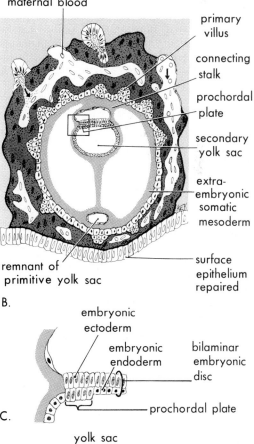

maternal blood

primary villus

connecting stalk

prochordal plate

secondary yolk sac

extra-embryonic somatic mesoderm

surface epithelium repaired

remnant of primitive yolk sac

B.

embryonic ectoderm

embryonic endoderm

bilaminar embryonic disc

prochordal plate

C.

yolk sac

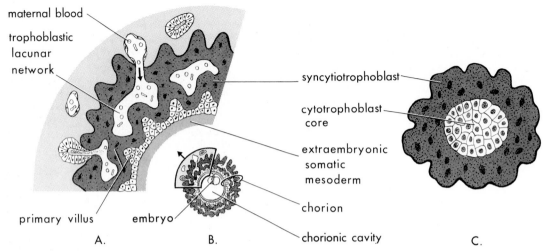

Figure 4–6. *A,* Detail of the section of the wall of the chorionic sac outlined in *B. B,* Sketch of a 14-day conceptus to illustrate the chorionic sac and the shaggy appearance created by the primary villi (×6). *C,* Drawing of a transverse section through a primary villus (×300).

The coelom splits the extraembryonic mesoderm into two layers (Fig. 4–5*A* and *B*): the *extraembryonic somatic mesoderm* lines the trophoblast and covers the amnion, and the *extraembryonic splanchnic mesoderm* covers the yolk sac. The extraembryonic somatic mesoderm and the trophoblast together constitute the chorion (Fig. 4–6*B*). The chorion forms a sac within which the embryo and its amnion and yolk sac are suspended by the connecting stalk. The amniotic sac (with the embryonic ectoderm forming its "floor") and the yolk sac (with the embryonic endoderm forming its "roof") are analogous to two balloons pressed together to form the embryonic disc and suspended by a cord (the connecting stalk) from the inside of a larger balloon (the chorionic sac).

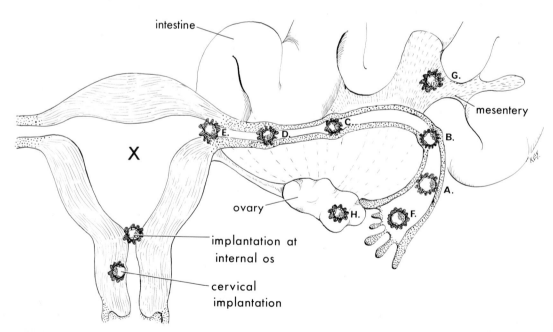

Figure 4–7. Drawing to illustrate various implantation sites; the usual site in the posterior wall is indicated by an X. The approximate order of frequency of ectopic (extrauterine) implantations is indicated alphabetically. *A* to *F,* Tubal pregnancies. *G,* Abdominal pregnancy. *H,* Ovarian pregnancy.

uterine tube   chorionic sac

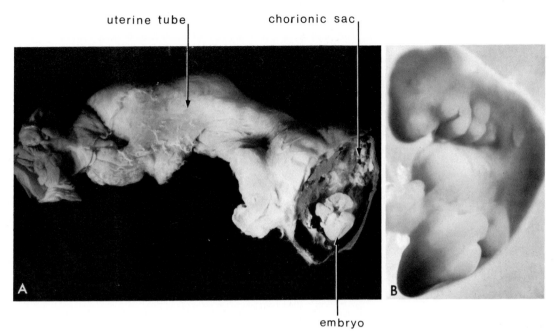

embryo

Figure 4–8. Photographs of a tubal pregnancy. *A,* The uterine tube has been sectioned to show the conceptus implanted in the mucous membrane (×3). *B,* Enlarged photograph of the normal-appearing four-week embryo (×13).

IMPLANTATION SITES

The blastocyst usually implants in the upper part of the uterus (Fig. 4–7). Implantation occasionally occurs outside the uterus, usually in the uterine tube; these are referred to as *ectopic implantations.* There are several causes of *tubal pregnancy,* but it is usually related to delayed transport of the dividing zygote to the uterus (Fig. 4–8). Ec-

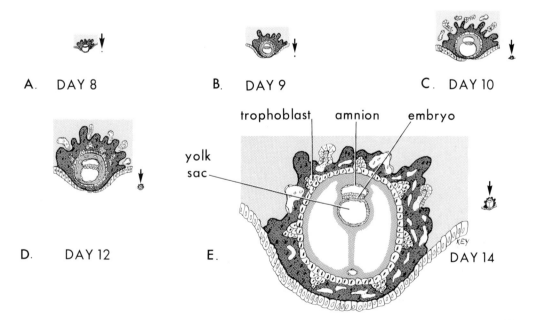

A.   DAY 8   B.   DAY 9   C.   DAY 10

trophoblast   amnion   embryo

yolk
sac

D.   DAY 12   E.   DAY 14

Figure 4–9. Drawings of sections of human blastocysts during the second week, illustrating the rapid expansion of the trophoblast and the relatively minute size of the embryos (×25); the sketches indicated by the arrows show the actual size of the blastocysts.

topic tubal pregnancies usually result in rupture and hemorrhage of the uterine tube during the first two months, and constitute a threat to the mother's life. Tubal rupture and expulsion of the embryo may be followed by a secondary implantation of the conceptus in the ovary (Fig. 4–7*H*) or in the abdomen (Fig. 4–7*G*). *Ovarian and abdominal pregnancies are extremely rare.* In exceptional cases an abdominal pregnancy progresses to full term and the fetus is delivered alive. Usually an abdominal pregnancy creates a serious condition because the placenta often attaches to vital structures and causes considerable bleeding.

Spontaneous Early Abortions

Most spontaneously aborted embryos recovered from women of known fertility are abnormal. About 25 per cent of early aborted embryos have chromosome abnormalities. Exposure of embryos to certain drugs during the first two weeks may kill them and cause early abortions (see Chapter 9).

SUMMARY

Rapid proliferation of the trophoblast occurs during the second week (Fig. 4–9). Lacunae develop in it and fuse to form *lacunar networks.* The trophoblast erodes maternal blood vessels and blood seeps into the lacunar networks, forming a primitive *uteroplacental circulation.* Primary *villi* form on the outer surface of the chorionic sac. Implantation is complete when the conceptus is wholly embedded within the endometrium and the surface epithelium grows over the embedded blastocyst.

Concurrently, extraembryonic mesoderm arises from the inner surface of the trophoblast and reduces the relative size of the blastocyst cavity, forming a primitive *yolk sac.* As the extraembryonic coelom forms from spaces in the extraembryonic mesoderm, the primitive yolk sac becomes smaller. The *amniotic cavity* appears as a slit-like space between the trophoblast and the inner cell mass. The inner cell mass differentiates into a *bilaminar embryonic disc* consisting of a layer of embryonic ectoderm and a layer of embryonic endoderm.

5

THE THIRD WEEK OF DEVELOPMENT

The third week is a period of rapid development of the embryo; it follows the first missed menstrual period (see Fig. 1–1). Cessation of menstruation is usually the first sign that a woman may be pregnant. Relatively simple and rapid tests are now available for detecting pregnancy. These tests depend on the presence of *human chorionic gonadotropin* (HCG), a hormone produced by the trophoblast and excreted in the mother's urine (see Chapter 8).

THE PRIMITIVE STREAK

Early in the third week, a thick linear band of embryonic ectoderm, known as the *primitive streak*, appears caudally in the midline of the dorsal aspect of the embryonic disc (Fig. 5–1A). As the primitive streak elongates by addition of cells at its caudal end (Fig. 5–2), its cranial end thickens to form a *primitive knot*. The primitive streak gives rise to mesenchymal cells which form loose embryonic connective tissue, often called *mesenchyme*.

By the sixteenth day the third primary germ layer, known as the *intraembryonic mesoderm*, begins to appear between the embryonic ectoderm and endoderm (Fig. 5–1B). Formation of this layer converts the bilaminar embryonic disc into a trilaminar, or three-layered, embryonic disc (Fig. 5–1E and F).

Cells migrate cranially from the primitive knot and form a midline cord known as the *notochordal process* (Figs. 5–1C and D and 5–

2B). This cord grows between the ectoderm and endoderm until it reaches the *prochordal plate*, which indicates the future site of the mouth. The notochordal process can extend no further because the prochordal plate is firmly attached to the overlying ectoderm, forming the *oropharyngeal membrane* (Figs. 5–2C and 5–3C). Caudal to the primitive streak a circular area forms which is known as the *cloacal membrane*. The embryonic disc remains bilaminar here also because the ectoderm and endoderm are fused (Fig. 5–3C).

Changes in the Embryonic Disc. Initially the embryonic disc is flat and essentially circular, but it soon becomes pear-shaped (Fig. 5–2A and B) and then elongated as the notochordal process grows (Fig. 5–2C and D). Expansion of the embryonic disc occurs mainly in the cranial region; the caudal end remains more or less unchanged. Much of the growth and elongation of the embryonic disc results from the continuous migration of mesenchymal cells from the primitive streak.

Fate of the Primitive Streak. The primitive streak continues to form mesenchyme until about the end of the fourth week; thereafter, mesenchyme production from this source slows down. The primitive streak quickly diminishes in relative size and becomes an insignificant structure in the sacrococcygeal region of the embryo (Fig. 5–2D). Normally it undergoes degenerative changes and disappears, but primitive streak remnants may persist and give rise to a tumor known as *teratoma*.

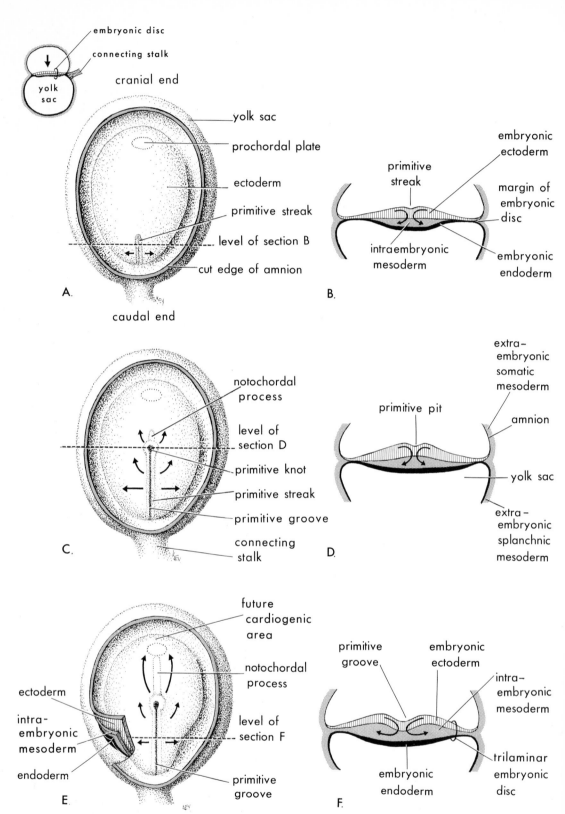

Figure 5–1. Drawings illustrating formation of the trilaminar embryonic disc (three-layered embryo). The small sketch at the upper left is for orientation; the arrow indicates the dorsal aspect of the embryonic disc as shown in A. The arrows in all other drawings indicate migration of mesenchymal cells between the ectoderm and endoderm. A, C and E, Dorsal views of the embryonic disc early in the third week, exposed by removal of the amnion. B, D and F, Transverse sections through the embryonic disc at the levels indicated.

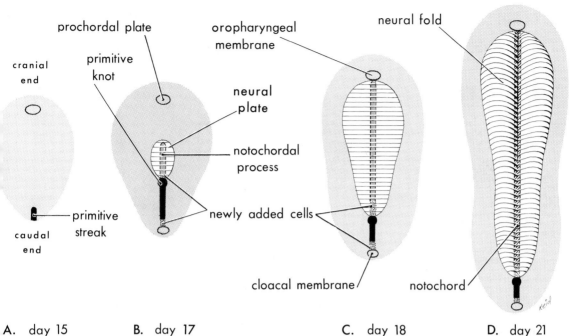

cranial end

prochordal plate

primitive knot

oropharyngeal membrane

neural fold

neural plate

notochordal process

primitive streak

newly added cells

caudal end

cloacal membrane

notochord

A. day 15   B. day 17   C. day 18   D. day 21

Figure 5–2. Sketches of dorsal views of the embryonic disc showing how it lengthens and changes shape during the third week. The primitive streak lengthens by addition of cells at its caudal end; the notochordal process lengthens by migration of cells from the primitive knot. The notochordal process and adjacent mesoderm induce the overlying embryonic ectoderm to form the neural plate, the primordium of the central nervous system.

The Notochord

The notochord is a cellular rod that develops from the notochordal process (Fig. 5–3). In a lower chordate, *Amphioxus*, the notochord forms the skeleton of the adult animal. This cellular rod forms a midline axis in the human embryo and the basis of the axial skeleton. The skull and vertebral column later develop around it and then it largely disappears (see Chapter 16).

THE NEURAL TUBE

As the notochord develops, the embryonic ectoderm over it and the adjacent mesoderm thickens to form the *neural plate* (Figs. 5–2B and 5–3A). This plate gives rise to the *central nervous system* (see Chapter 17). The neural plate first appears cranial to the primitive knot, but as the notochordal process elongates, the neural plate broadens and eventually extends cranially as far as the *oropharyngeal membrane* (Fig. 5–2C). On about the eighteenth day, the neural plate invaginates along its central axis to form a

neural groove with neural folds on each side (Figs. 5–2D and 5–4A and B). By the end of the third week, the *neural folds* at the middle of the embryo have moved together and fused, converting the neural plate into a *neural tube* (Fig. 5–4F).

The Allantois

The allantois (from Greek *allantos,* meaning "sausage") appears early in the third week as a relatively small, finger-like outpouching or diverticulum from the caudal wall of the yolk sac (Fig. 5–3B). The allantois remains very small in the human embryo, but it is involved with early blood and blood vessel formation and is associated with development of the urinary bladder (see Chapter 14).

DEVELOPMENT OF SOMITES

By the end of the third week, the mesoderm beside the neural tube and the notochord, called the *paraxial mesoderm,* begins

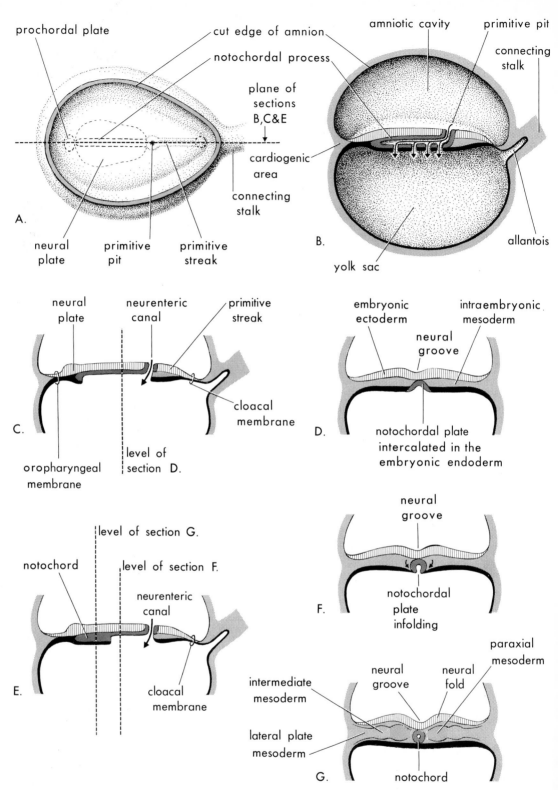

Figure 5–3. Drawings illustrating notochord development. *A*, Dorsal view of the embryonic disc at about 18 days, exposed by removing the amnion. *B*, Three-dimensional sagittal section of the embryo, showing the numerous openings in the floor of the notochordal process which temporarily permit communication between the amniotic cavity and the yolk sac. *C* and *E*, Sagittal sections of embryos of about 18 to 19 days. *D*, *F*, and *G*, Transverse sections of the embryonic disc. Note that the notochordal plate, formed from the notochordal process, infolds to form the notochord.

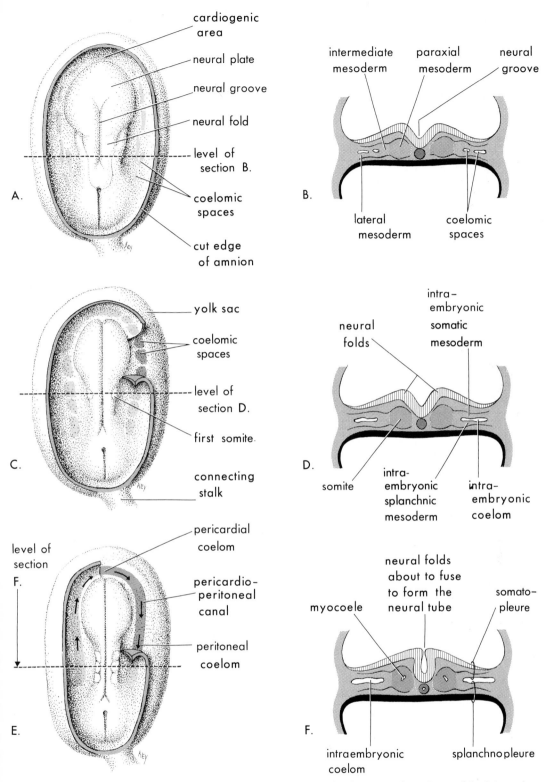

Figure 5—4. Drawings of embryos of 19 to 21 days, illustrating development of somites and the intraembryonic coelom. *A, C* and *E,* Dorsal views of the embryonic disc, exposed by removal of the amnion. *B, D* and *F,* Transverse sections through the embryonic disc at the levels shown. *A,* Presomite embryo of about 19 days. *C,* An embryo of about 20 days showing the first pair of somites. A portion of the ectoderm and mesoderm on the right side has been removed to show the coelomic spaces in the lateral plate mesoderm. *E,* A three-somite embryo of about 21 days showing the horseshoe-shaped intraembryonic coelom, exposed on the right by removal of the ectoderm and mesoderm of the embryo.

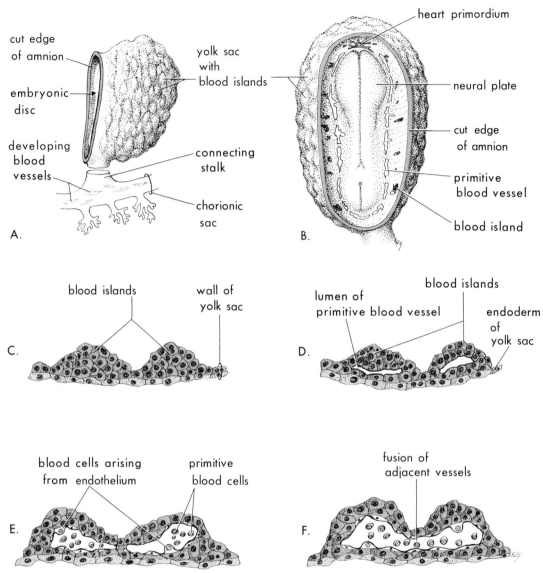

Figure 5–5. Successive stages in the development of blood and blood vessels. *A,* The yolk sac and a portion of the chorionic sac at about 18 days. *B,* Dorsal view of an embryo of about 19 days, exposed by removing the amnion. *C* to *F,* Sections of blood islands showing progressive stages of development of blood and blood vessels.

to divide into paired cuboidal bodies called *somites* (Fig. 5–4*C* and *D*). The first pair of somites develops a short distance caudal to the cranial end of the notochord, and subsequent pairs form in a craniocaudal sequence. About 38 pairs of somites form during the so-called somite period (days 20 to 30); eventually 42 to 44 pairs develop. The somites form distinct surface elevations (Fig. 5–4*E*) and are somewhat triangular in transverse section. A transitory slit-like cavity, the *myocoele,* appears within each somite

(Fig. 5–6*F*). The word somite is from the Greek *soma,* meaning "a body." The somites give rise to most of the axial skeleton and associated musculature as well as much of the dermis of the skin (see Chapters 16 and 19).

DEVELOPMENT OF THE COELOM

The intraembryonic coelom or embryonic body cavity first appears as a number of isolated *coelomic spaces* within the lateral mesoderm and the mesoderm that will form the heart, called the cardiogenic mesoderm (Fig. 5–4*A* and *B*). These spaces soon coalesce to form a horseshoe-shaped cavity, the *intraembryonic coelom* (Fig. 5–4*E*).

The intraembryonic coelom divides the lateral plate mesoderm into two layers (Fig. 5–4*D*): a *somatic (parietal) layer* continuous with the extraembryonic mesoderm covering the amnion, and a *splanchnic (visceral) layer* continuous with the extraembryonic mesoderm covering the yolk sac. The somatic mesoderm and the overlying embryonic ectoderm form the body wall or *somatopleure* (Fig. 5–4*F*), whereas the splanchnic mesoderm and the embryonic endoderm form the *splanchnopleure* or wall of the future primitive gut.

During the second month, the intraembryonic coelom is divided into three body cavities (see Chapter 10): (1) the *pericardial cavity* containing the heart, (2) the *pleural cavities* containing the lungs, and (3) the *peri-toneal cavity* containing the viscera lying caudal to the diaphragm.

PRIMITIVE CARDIOVASCULAR SYSTEM

Blood vessel formation begins early in the third week in the extraembryonic mesoderm of the yolk sac, connecting stalk and chorion. Embryonic vessels develop about two days later. The early formation of the cardiovascular system is correlated with the absence of a significant amount of yolk in the ovum and yolk sac. Consequently, there is a need for vessels to bring nourishment and oxygen to the embryo from the maternal circulation.

Blood and blood vessel formation may be summarized as follows: (1) mesenchymal cells aggregate to form isolated masses and cords known as *blood islands* (Fig. 5–5*A* to *C*);

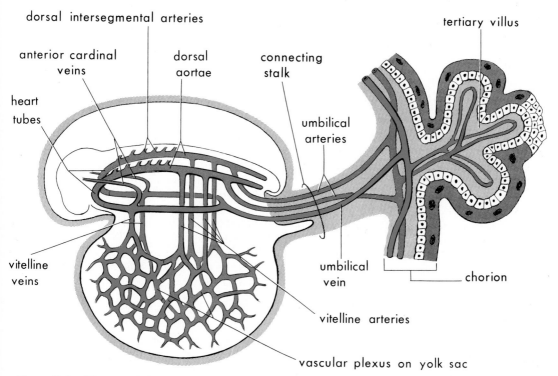

Figure 5–6. Diagram of the primitive cardiovascular system in a 21-day embryo viewed from the left side, showing the transitory stage of paired symmetrical vessels. Each heart tube continues dorsally into a *dorsal aorta* which passes caudally; branches of the aortae are: (1) *umbilical arteries*, establishing connections with vessels in the chorion, (2) *vitelline arteries* to the yolk sac, and (3) *dorsal intersegmental arteries* to the body of the embryo. An *umbilical vein* returns blood from the chorion and divides into right and left umbilical veins within the embryo. Vessels on the yolk sac form a *vascular plexus* which is connected to the heart by *vitelline veins*. The *anterior cardinal veins* return blood from the head region.

(2) spaces appear within these islands (Fig. 5–5*D*); (3) cells arrange themselves around the cavity to form the primitive *endothelium* (Fig. 5–5*E*); (4) isolated vessels fuse to form networks of endothelial channels (Fig. 5–5*F*); and (5) vessels extend into adjacent areas by fusing with other vessels formed independently.

Primitive plasma and blood cells develop from the endothelial cells of the vessels (Fig. 5–5*E*). Blood formation does not begin within the embryo until the second month, where it first occurs in the liver and later in the spleen, bone marrow and lymph nodes. Mesenchymal cells surrounding the primitive endothelial vessels differentiate into the muscular and connective tissue elements of the vessels.

The primitive heart tubes form in a similar manner from mesenchymal cells in the *cardiogenic area* (Fig. 5–5*B*). Paired *heart tubes* develop before the end of the third week and begin to fuse into the primitive heart tube. By the twenty-first day, the paired heart tubes have linked up with blood vessels in the embryo, connecting stalk, chorion and yolk sac to form a primitive cardiovascular system (Fig. 5–6). The circulation of blood has almost certainly started by the end of the third week, and so *the cardiovascular system is the first organ system to reach a functional state.*

SUMMARY

As the intraembryonic mesoderm forms, the bilaminar embryonic disc is converted into a trilaminar embryo composed of three *primary germ layers* (ectoderm, mesoderm and endoderm). These layers will later give rise to all tissues and organs in the embryo.

The *primitive streak* appears early in the third week as a midline thickening of the embryonic ectoderm. It gives rise to mesenchymal cells which migrate laterally and cranially between the ectoderm and endoderm, and organize into the third primary germ layer, the intraembryonic mesoderm. The primitive knot gives rise to the *notochordal process*. The *notochord* develops from the notochordal process and forms the primitive skeletal support of the embryo.

The *neural plate* appears as a midline thickening of the embryonic ectoderm, cranial to the primitive knot. A longitudinal *neural groove* develops which is flanked by *neural folds;* these folds meet and fuse to form the *neural tube.*

The mesoderm on each side of the no- tochord thickens to form longitudinal columns of *paraxial mesoderm*. Division of the paraxial mesoderm into pairs of *somites* begins cranially by the end of the third week. The intraembryonic coelom arises as isolated spaces in the *lateral plate mesoderm* and *cardiogenic mesoderm*. These coelomic spaces subsequently coalesce to form a single, horseshoe-shaped cavity which eventually gives rise to the body cavities.

Blood vessels first appear on the yolk sac, the allantois and in the chorion and develop within the embryo shortly thereafter. Spaces appear within aggregations of mesenchyme (*blood islands*) which soon become lined with endothelium and unite with other spaces to form a primitive cardiovascular system. At the end of the third week, the heart is represented by paired *heart tubes* which are joined to blood vessels in the extraembryonic membranes. The primitive blood cells are derived mainly from the endothelial cells of blood vessels in the yolk sac and allantois.

6

THE FOURTH TO SEVENTH WEEKS

The rapidity of embryonic development during the fourth to seventh weeks is amazing. The beginnings of all major external and internal structures develop during this so-called *embryonic period.* Exposure of an embryo to certain agents (drugs, viruses, etc.) during this *critical period of development* may cause major congenital malformations (see Chapter 9).

FOLDING OF THE EMBRYO

During the fourth week, the embryo grows rapidly (tripling its size) and its shape changes significantly as the result of folding. The gradual establishment of body form largely results from folding of the flat embryonic disc into a somewhat cylindrical embryo. This infolding in both longitudinal and transverse planes is mainly caused by rapid growth of the neural tube. The formation of longitudinal and transverse folds is a simultaneous process of constriction at the junction of the embryo and yolk sac and not a separate sequence of events. Folding in the longitudinal plane produces head and tail folds that result in the cranial and caudal regions "swinging" ventrally as if on a hinge (Fig. $6-1A_2$ to D_2). During folding, part of the yolk sac is incorporated into the embryo.

The Head Fold. The brain grows cranially beyond the oropharyngeal membrane and soon overhangs the primitive heart. The heart and oropharyngeal membrane also turn under onto the ventral surface. After folding, the mass of mesoderm cranial to the pericardial coelom, called the *septum transversum,* lies caudal to the heart. Subsequently, this septum develops into a major part of the diaphragm (see Chapter 10).

The Tail Fold. Folding of the caudal end occurs a little later than that of the cranial end (Fig. $6-1C_2$). As the embryo grows, the tail region projects over the *cloacal membrane.* The *connecting stalk* later attaches to the ventral surface of the embryo.

Transverse Folding. Folding of the embryo in the transverse plane produces right and left *lateral folds* (Fig. $6-1A_3$ to D_3). Each lateral body wall folds toward the midline, rolling the edges of the embryonic disc ventrally and forming a roughly cylindrical embryo. As the lateral and ventral body walls form, part of the yolk sac is incorporated into the embryo as the *midgut* (Fig. $6-1D_2$ and D_3). Concurrently, the connection of the midgut with the yolk sac is reduced to a narrow *yolk stalk* or vitelline duct (Fig. $6-1C_2$). After folding, the region of the attachment of the amnion to the embryo is reduced to a relatively narrow region, the *umbilicus,* on the ventral surface (Fig. $6-1D_2$). As the midgut is separated from the yolk sac, it becomes attached to the dorsal abdominal wall by a thin *dorsal mesentery* (Fig. $6-1D_3$). As the amniotic cavity expands and obliterates the extraembryonic coelom, the amnion forms an external investment for the *umbilical cord* (Fig. $6-1D_2$). Development of the umbilical cord is also discussed in Chapter 8.

CONTROL OF DEVELOPMENT

The three primary germ layers (ectoderm, mesoderm and endoderm) give rise to all tissues and organs of the embryo (Fig. 6-2). Development results from genetic

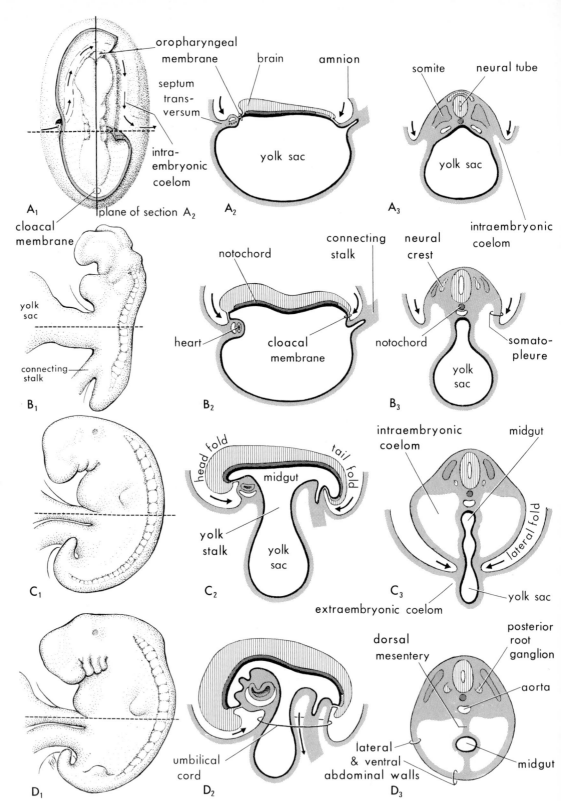

Figure 6–1. Drawings of four-week embryos illustrating folding in both longitudinal and transverse planes. A_1, Dorsal view of a 22-day embryo. The continuity of the intraembryonic coelom and extraembryonic coelom is illustrated on the right side by removal of a portion of the embryonic ectoderm and mesoderm. B_1, C_1 and D_1, Lateral views of embryos of about 24, 26 and 28 days, respectively. A_2 to D_2, Longitudinal sections at the plane shown in A_1. A_3 to D_3, Transverse sections at the levels indicated in A_1 to D_1.

44

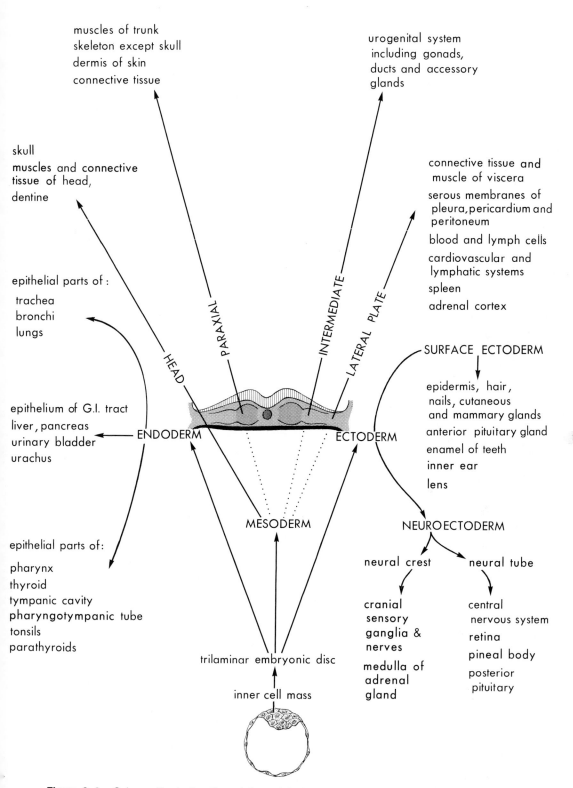

Figure 6–2. Scheme illustrating the origin and derivatives of the three primary germ layers.

plans contained in the chromosomes. The individuality of each person is largely determined at fertilization by the genes contained in the chromosomes of the sperm and the ovum. These genes control the processes by which the body develops before and after birth. Defective genetic plans (abnormal number of chromosomes, gene mutations and so forth) result in maldevelopment. Abnormal development may also be caused by environmental factors (discussed in Chapter 9). Most developmental processes depend upon a precisely coordinated interaction of genetic and environmental factors. There are several control mechanisms that guide differentiation and insure synchronized development.

Induction

For a limited time during early development, certain embryonic tissues markedly influence the development of adjacent tissues. The tissues producing these influences or effects are called *inductors* or organizers. Induction involves two tissues: the inducting tissue or inductor, and the induced tissue. In order to induce, an inductor must be close to but not necessarily in contact with, the tissue to be induced. In birds, and probably in humans, the primitive streak, notochordal process and paraxial mesoderm act as primary organizers of the central nervous system (Fig. 6–3).

Once the basic embryonic plan has been

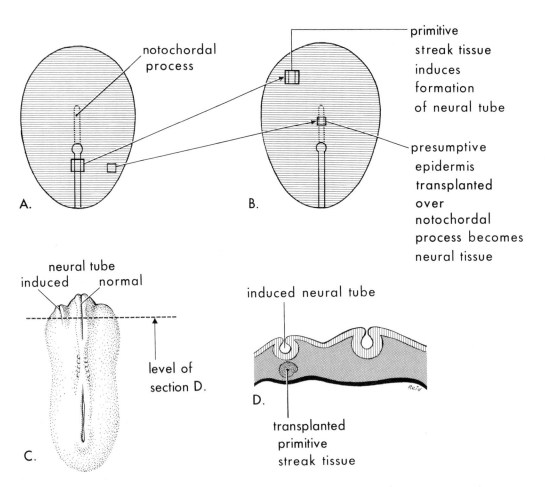

Figure 6–3. *A* and *B,* Dorsal views of avian embryonic discs illustrating experimental induction of the neural tube. *C,* Dorsal view of an embryo showing a normal and an induced neural tube. *D,* Transverse section through the embryo at the level shown, illustrating the secondary neural tube which was induced by the transplanted piece of primitive streak.

established by primary organizers, a chain of *secondary inductions* occurs. The nature of the inductive agents is not clearly understood, but it is generally accepted that some substance passes from the inducing tissue to the induced tissue.

HIGHLIGHTS OF THE EMBRYONIC PERIOD

The following descriptions summarize the main developmental events and changes in external form. The details of organ formation are given with discussions of the various systems (Chapters 12 to 19).

The Fourth Week. Initially, the embryo is almost straight and the *somites* (precursors of muscles and vertebrae) produce conspicuous surface elevations (Fig. 6–4*A* and *B*). The neural tube is closed opposite the somites but is widely open at rostral and caudal openings called *neuropores.* By 24 days the first (or mandibular) and the second (or hyoid) *branchial arches* are visible (Fig. 6–4*C*). The major portion, or mandibular process, of the first arch forms the lower jaw, and an extension of it, the maxillary process, contributes to the upper jaw (see Chapter 11). A slight curve is produced in the embryo by the head and tail folds, and the heart produces a large ventral prominence. Three branchial arches are visible by 26 days (Figs. 6–4*D* and 6–5), and the forebrain produces a prominent elevation on the head. Continued longitudinal folding has given the

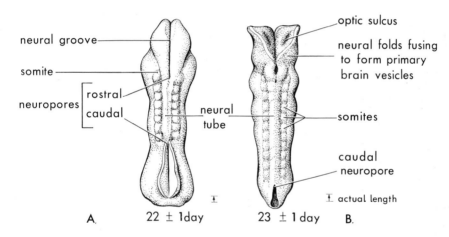

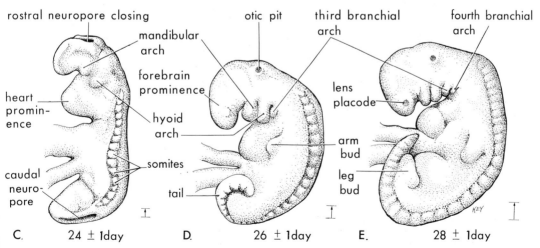

Figure 6–4. Drawings of four-week embryos. *A* and *B,* Dorsal views of embryos with 8 and 12 somites, respectively. *C, D* and *E,* Lateral views of embryos with 16, 27 and 33 somites, respectively.

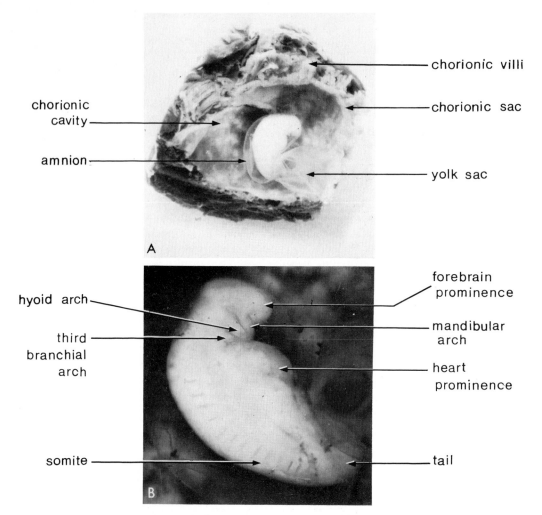

chorionic villi

chorionic sac

chorionic cavity

amnion

yolk sac

A

forebrain prominence

hyoid arch

mandibular arch

third branchial arch

heart prominence

somite

tail

B

Figure 6–5. *A*, Photograph of a four-week embryo in the amniotic sac, exposed by opening the chorionic sac (×5). *B*, Higher magnification of the embryo of about 26 days (×18). For a discussion of the branchial arches and other parts of the branchial apparatus, see Chapter 11.

embryo a characteristic C-shaped curvature. The *arm buds* become recognizable as small swellings on the lateral body walls (Fig. 6–4D). The *otic pits*, the primordia of the inner ears, are also clearly visible. The *leg buds* are present by 28 days (Fig. 6–4E). Lens placodes, ectodermal thickenings indicating the future lenses, are visible on the sides of the head.

The Fifth Week. Changes in body form are minor compared with the fourth week. Extensive head growth is caused mainly by the rapid development of the brain (Figs. 6–6 and 6–7). The limbs show considerable regional differentiation, especially the forelimbs. The elbow and wrist regions become identifiable, and the paddle-shaped hand

plates develop digital ridges, called *finger* or *digital rays*, indicating the future fingers (Fig. 6–6C). Note that development of the hindlimb occurs somewhat later than that of the forelimb.

Several small swellings develop around the groove between the first two branchial arches; this groove becomes the *external acoustic meatus*, and the swellings eventually fuse to form the auricle (external ear).

The Sixth Week. The head is now much larger relative to the trunk, and is more bent over the *heart prominence* (Figs. 6–8 and 6–9). This head position results from bending of the brain in the cervical region. By 42 days the somites are no longer visible. The intestines enter the extraembryonic coelom in

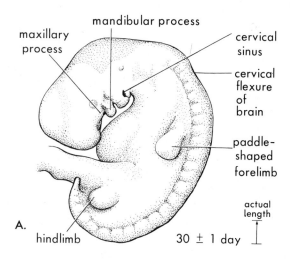

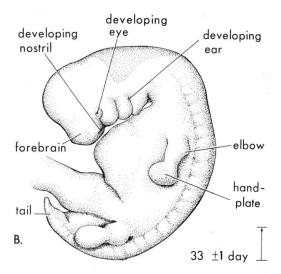

Figure 6–6. Drawings of lateral views of five-week embryos.

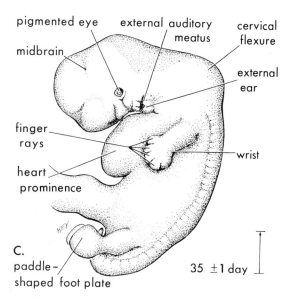

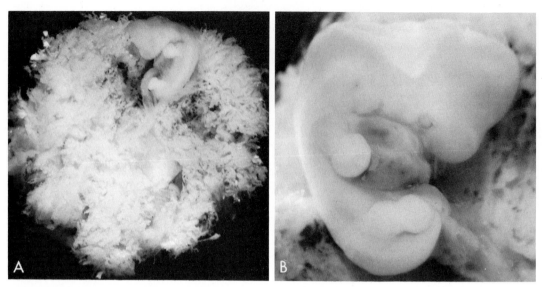

Figure 6–7. *A*, Photograph of a five-week embryo in the amniotic sac, exposed by opening the chorionic sac (×2). *B*, Higher magnification of the embryo of about 35 days (×6). Compare with Figure 6–6 *C*.

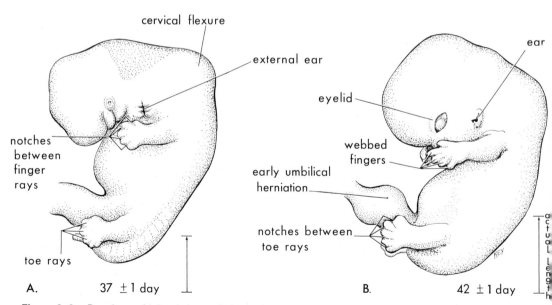

Figure 6–8. Drawings of lateral views of six-week embryos.

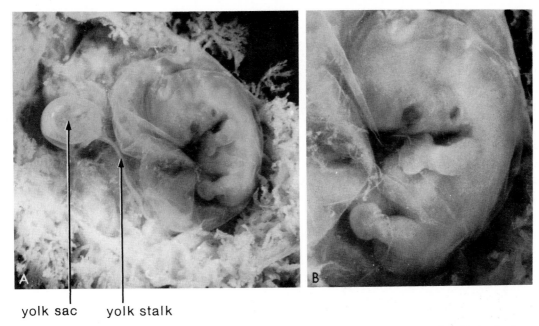

yolk sac   yolk stalk

Figure 6–9. *A*, Photograph of a six-week embryo in the amniotic sac, exposed by opening the chorionic sac (×2.8). *B*, Higher magnification of the embryo of about 36 days (×5). Note the low position of the ear at this stage.

the proximal portion of the umbilical cord. The communication between the primitive gut and the yolk sac is now reduced to a relatively small *yolk stalk* (Fig. 6–9*A*).

The limbs undergo considerable change during the sixth week. By 42 days they have lengthened and flexed slightly so that the fingers reach the nose (Fig. 6–8*B*). Notches appear between the rays in the hand plates, indicating the future fingers. Short, webbed fingers are soon present and notches appear between the toe rays in the foot plates (Figs. 6–8*B* and 6–10*B*).

The Seventh Week. The embryo now has unquestionably human characteristics (Figs. 6–11*B* and 6–12). The head is more rounded and erect, but it is still disproportionately large. The neck region has become established and the eyelids are more obvious. The forearms gradually rise above the shoulder level, and the hands often cover the mouth and nose regions. The fingers and toes are well differentiated. The abdomen is less protuberant, but the intestine is still in the umbilical cord (Fig. 6–12).

ESTIMATION OF EMBRYONIC AGE

Information about the starting date of pregnancies may be unreliable, partly be-cause it depends on the mother's memory. Two reference points are commonly used for estimating age: the onset of the last menstrual period (LMP), and the time of fertilization. The probability of error in establishing the last normal menses is highest in women who become pregnant after discontinuing oral contraceptives. This is because the interval between stopping the hormones and ovulation is highly variable. In addition, vaginal bleeding or "spotting" sometimes occurs after implantation of the blastocyst and is incorrectly regarded as menstruation.

It must be emphasized that the zygote does not form until about two weeks after LMP (the onset of the last menstrual period, see Fig. 1–1). Consequently, 13 ± 1 days must be deducted from the menstrual age to obtain the actual or *fertilization age* of an embryo. The day fertilization occurs is the most accurate reference point for estimating age. This is commonly calculated from the estimated time of ovulation because the ovum is usually fertilized within 12 hours after ovulation.

Because it may be important to know the actual or fertilization age of an embryo, e.g., for determining its sensitivity to drugs (Chapter 9), all statements about age should indicate the reference point used, i.e., weeks after LMP or fertilization. Estimates

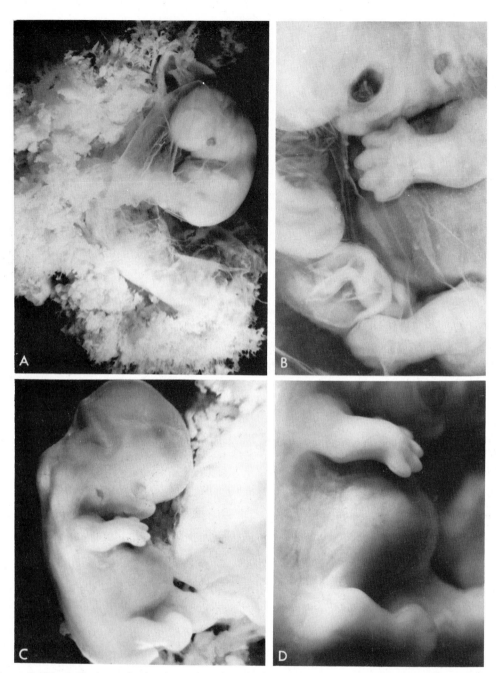

Figure 6–10. *A*, Photograph of a six-week embryo in the amniotic sac, exposed by opening the chorionic sac (×2). *B*, Higher magnification of this embryo of about 38 days (×7). *C*, Photograph of a slightly older six-week embryo, exposed by removal from the chorionic and amniotic sacs (×4). *D*, Higher magnification of this embryo of about 39 days (×7). The large abdominal prominence is caused mainly by the liver; most of the intestine is in the umbilical cord.

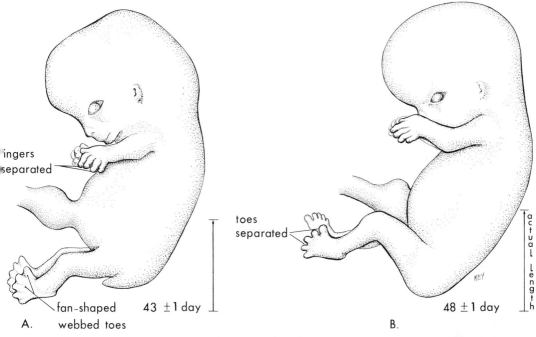

fingers
separated

toes
separated

fan-shaped
webbed toes

A.

43 ±1 day

48 ±1 day

actual length

KEY

B.

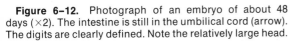

Figure 6–11. Drawings of lateral views of seven-week embryos.

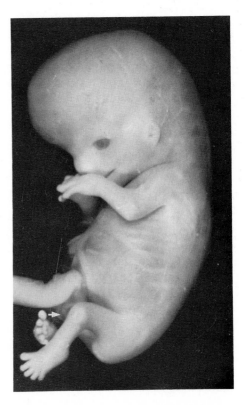

Figure 6–12. Photograph of an embryo of about 48 days (×2). The intestine is still in the umbilical cord (arrow). The digits are clearly defined. Note the relatively large head.

TABLE 6–1. CRITERIA FOR ESTIMATING FERTILIZATION AGE DURING THE EMBRYONIC PERIOD

Age ±1 Day	No. of Somites	Crown-Rump Length (mm)	Main External Characteristics
22	4–12	1.5–2.0	*Embryo essentially straight.* Neural folds fused opposite somites.
24	13–20	2.0–3.0	*Embryo slightly curved.* Two branchial arches visible.
26	21–29	3.0–3.5	*Embryo C-shaped.* Three branchial arches visible. Forebrain produces prominence. Arm buds appear as small swellings. Otic pits present.
28	33–35	4.0–5.0	*Four branchial arches visible.* Caudal neuropore closed. Flipper-like arm bud. Leg bud appears as small swelling. Lens placode visible.
30	36–38	6.0–7.0	*Forelimb paddle-shaped;* hindlimb flipper-like. Third and fourth arches at the bottom of cervical sinus.
33	*	8.0–10.0	*Hand plate formed;* hindlimb paddle-shaped. Wrist and elbow visible. Definite eye and nostril.
35		12.0–14.0	*Finger rays in hand plate;* foot plate formed. Ear swellings present. Pigment in eye. Prominent tail.
37		14.6–15.6	*Notches between finger rays* in hand plate; toe rays in foot plate. Distinct cervical flexure.
40		21.0–22.0	*Notches between toe rays;* stubby fingers. Eyelids visible.
42		23.0–23.5	*Fingers short and slightly webbed.* Fingertips swollen. Intestine causes swelling in umbilical cord. Stubby tail.
45		25.0–27.0	*Toes short and slightly webbed.* Fingers elongated.
48		28.0–30.0	*Digits of both hands and feet clearly defined.* Head, trunk and limbs have human characteristics. Tail absent.

*At this and subsequent stages, the number of somites is not a useful criterion for estimating age.

of the age of recovered embryos (e. g., after abortion) are determined from external characteristics and measurements of length (Table 6–1). The changing appearance of the developing limbs is also a very useful criterion. Size alone may be an unreliable criterion because some embryos probably undergo a progressively slower rate of growth prior to death.

Methods of Measurement. Because em-

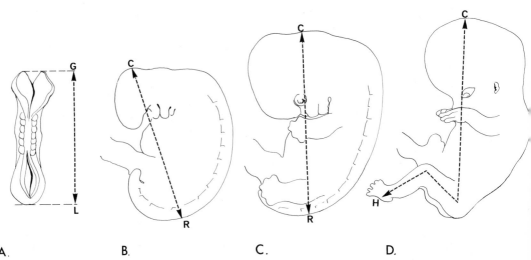

A.   B.   C.   D.

Figure 6–13. Sketches showing methods of measuring the length of embryos. *A,* Greatest length. *B* and *C,* Crown-rump length. *D,* Crown-heel length.

bryos of the third and early fourth weeks are nearly straight, measurements indicate the *greatest length* (GL, Fig. 6–13*A*). The sitting height or *crown-rump length* (CR, Fig. 6– 13*B* and *C*) is most frequently used for older embryos. Standing height or *crown-heel length* (CH, Fig. 6–13*D*) is sometimes used for seven-week and older specimens.

SUMMARY

Early in the embryonic period, longitudinal and transverse folding converts the flat trilaminar embryonic disc into a C-shaped cylindrical embryo. The dorsal part of the yolk sac is incorporated into the embryo during folding and gives rise to the *primitive gut.* The gut becomes pinched off from the yolk sac but remains attached to it by the narrow *yolk stalk.* As the amnion expands, it forms an external investment for the *umbilical cord.* The head fold results in the heart coming to lie ventrally and the brain becoming the most cranial part of the embryo. The tail fold causes the connecting stalk (future umbilical cord) and allantois to move to the ventral surface of the embryo.

By the end of the embryonic period, the beginnings of all the main organ systems have been established. The embryo has characteristics which mark it as unquestionably human. *These four weeks constitute the most critical period of development.* Developmental disturbances during this period may give rise to major congenital malformations.

7

THE EIGHTH WEEK TO BIRTH

At about eight weeks the embryo is referred to as a fetus,[1] signifying that it has developed into a recognizable human being. In addition the fetus is far less vulnerable than the embryo to the deforming effects of drugs, viruses and radiation (see Chapter 9).

Development during the fetal period is primarily concerned with growth and maturation of tissues and organs that appeared during the embryonic period. Very few new structures appear during the fetal period.

---

[1]Latin word meaning offspring.

The rate of body growth is remarkable, especially between the twelfth and sixteenth weeks (Figs. 7–1 and 7–4), and weight gain is phenomenal during the terminal months (see Table 7–2 and Fig. 7–11).

ESTIMATION OF FETAL AGE

Pregnancy or the gestational period may be divided into days, weeks or months (Table 7–1). Confusion arises if it is not stated whether a given time is calculated

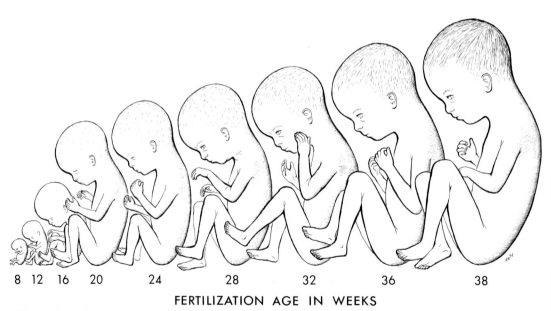

8 12 16   20   24   28   32   36   38

FERTILIZATION AGE IN WEEKS

Figure 7–1. Drawings of fetuses, about *one-fifth actual size.* Head hair begins to appear at about 20 weeks. Eyebrows and eyelashes are usually recognizable by 24 weeks, and the eyes reopen by 28 weeks.

TABLE 7-1. COMPARISON OF GESTATIONAL TIME UNITS

Reference Point	Days	Weeks	Calendar Months	Lunar Months
Fertilization*	266	38	8¾	9½
Last Menstrual Period	280	40	9	10

*The date of birth is calculated as about 266 days after fertilization, or 280 days after the onset of the last normal menstrual period. From fertilization to the end of the embryonic period, age is best expressed in days; thereafter age is commonly given in weeks. Because ovulation and fertilization are usually separated by not more than 12 hours, these events are more or less interchangeable in expressing prenatal age.

from the onset of the last menstrual period (LMP), or from the estimated day of ovulation or fertilization. More uncertainty arises when months are used, particularly when it is not stated whether calendar months (28 to 31 days) or lunar *months* (28 days) are meant. Unless otherwise stated, age in this book is calculated from estimated time of fertilization, and months refer to calendar months. *It is best to express fetal age in weeks*

TABLE 7-2. CRITERIA FOR ESTIMATING FERTILIZATION AGE DURING THE FETAL PERIOD

Age (weeks)	CR Length (mm)*	Foot Length (mm)*	Fetal Weight (gm)†	Main External Characteristics
A. *PREVIABLE FETUSES*				
8	40	6	5	*Eyes open.* Low-set ears. Short neck. Intestine in umbilical cord.
9	50	7	8	*Eyes closing or closed.* Head more rounded. External genitalia still not distinguishable as male or female.
10	61	9	14	*Intestine in abdomen.* Early fingernail development.
12	87	14	45	*Sex distinguishable externally.* Well-defined neck.
14	120	20	110	*Head erect.* Hindlimbs well developed.
16	140	27	200	*Ears stand out* from head.
18	160	33	320	*Vernix caseosa present.* Early toenail development.
20	190	39	460	*Head and body (lanugo) hair visible.*
22	210	45	630	*Skin wrinkled* and red.
24	230	50	820	*Fingernails present.* Lean body.
B. *VIABLE FETUSES‡*				
26	250	55	1000	*Eyes partially open.* Eyelashes present.
28	270	59	1300	*Eyes open.* Good head of hair. Skin slightly wrinkled.
30	280	63	1700	*Toenails present.* Body filling out.
32	300	68	2100	*Fingernails reach finger tips.* Skin pink and smooth.
36	340	79	2900	*Body usually plump.* Lanugo hairs almost absent. Toenails reach toe tips.
38	360	83	3400	*Prominent chest*; mammary glands protrude. Testes in scrotum or palpable in inguinal canals. Fingernails extend beyond finger tips.

*These measurements are averages and so may not apply to specific cases; dimensional variations increase with age. The method for taking CR (crown-rump) measurements is illustrated in Figure 6–13.

†These weights refer to fetuses that have been fixed for about two weeks in 10 per cent formalin. Fresh specimens usually weigh about five per cent less.

‡There is no sharp limit of development, age or weight at which a fetus automatically becomes viable or beyond which survival is assured, but experience has shown that it is unusual for a baby to survive whose weight is less than 1000 gm or whose fertilization age is less than 26 weeks.

and to state whether the beginning or the end of a week is meant.

Clinically, gestation is commonly divided into three parts, or *trimesters*, each lasting three calendar months. By the end of the first trimester, all major systems are developed and the crown-rump length of the fetus is about the width of one's palm. At the end of the second trimester, the fetus is still unable to survive independently, even though its length is now equal to about the span of one's hand.

Accurate determination of fetal age may not be possible for the reasons discussed in Chapter 6, but various measurements and external characteristics are useful in *estimating fetal age* (Table 7–2). *Foot length* correlates well with CR length and is particularly useful for estimating the age of incomplete or macerated fetuses. *Fetal weight* is often a useful criterion, but there may be a discrepancy between the fertilization age and the weight of a fetus, particularly when the mother has had metabolic disturbances during pregnancy; e.g., in diabetes mellitus, fetal weight often exceeds values considered normal for the length.

HIGHLIGHTS OF THE FETAL PERIOD

Eight to Twelve Weeks. At the beginning of the eighth week, the head constitutes almost half the fetus (Fig. 7–2). Thereafter, growth in body length accelerates rapidly so that by the end of 12 weeks fetal length has more than doubled (Table 7–2). Growth of the head slows down considerably, however, compared with the rest of the body. The face is broad, the eyes widely separated, and the ears low-set. At the beginning of the ninth week, the legs are short and the thighs are relatively small (Fig. 7–3). At the end of 12 weeks, the upper limbs have almost reached their final relative lengths, but the lower limbs are still not so well developed and are slightly shorter than their final relative length (Fig. 7–2). *The external genitalia of males and females appear somewhat similar until the end of the ninth week,* and their mature form is not established until the twelfth week (see Chapter 14). Intestinal coils are visible within the proximal end of the umbilical cord (Fig. 7–3B) until the middle of the tenth week.

Thirteen to Sixteen Weeks. Growth is very

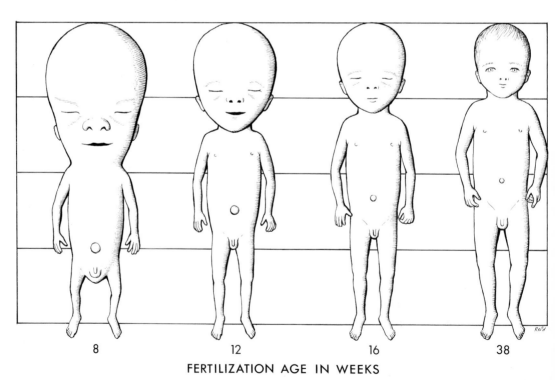

8   12   16   38

FERTILIZATION AGE IN WEEKS

Figure 7–2. Diagram illustrating the changing proportions of the body during the fetal period. All stages are drawn to the same total height. (Based on Scammon and Calkins, 1929.)

chorionic villi   amniotic sac

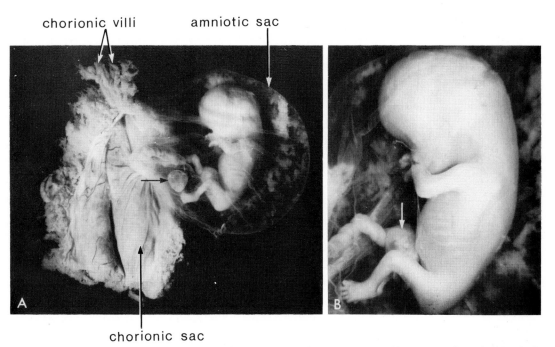

chorionic sac

Figure 7–3. Photographs of a nine-week fetus in the amniotic sac exposed by removal from the chorionic sac. *A, Actual size.* The remnant of the yolk sac is indicated by an arrow. *B,* Enlarged photograph of the fetus (×2). Note the following features: (1) large head, (2) cartilaginous ribs and (3) intestine in the umbilical cord (arrow).

rapid during this period (Table 7–2 and Fig. 7–4). At the end of this period, the head is relatively small compared with that of the 11-week fetus (Fig. 7–5), and the legs have lengthened (Fig. 7–6). The skeleton shows clearly on X-ray films toward the end of this period.

Seventeen to Twenty Weeks. Growth slows down during this period (Table 7–2). Fetal movements (known as *quickening*) are commonly recognized by the mother. The skin is covered with a greasy cheese-like material known as *vernix caseosa* (Fig. 7–7). It consists of a mixture of a fatty secretion from the fetal sebaceous glands and dead skin (see Chapter 19); it protects the fetus' delicate skin from abrasions, chapping and hardening as a result of being bathed in amniotic fluid. Twenty-week fetuses are usually completely covered with fine downy hair called *lanugo;* this may help hold the vernix on the skin. Eyebrows and head hair are also visible at the end of this period.

Twenty-one to Twenty-five Weeks. There is a substantial weight gain during this period. Although the body is still somewhat lean, it is better proportioned (Fig. 7–8).

The skin is usually wrinkled and is pink to red in color because blood in the capillaries is now visible.

Twenty-six to Twenty-nine Weeks. A fetus could now survive if born prematurely (Table 7–2), but the mortality rate is high, usually because of respiratory difficulty. The fetus is able to survive mainly because its central nervous system has matured so that it can direct rhythmic breathing and control body temperature. The eyes reopen during this period, and head and lanugo hair are well developed (Fig. 7–9). The fetus usually assumes an upside-down position as the time of birth approaches; this positioning results partly from the shape of the uterus and partly because the head is heavier than the feet.

Thirty to Thirty-eight Weeks. Most fetuses during this "finishing" period are plump (Fig. 7–10). Generally there is a slowing of growth as the time of birth approaches (Fig. 7–11). By full term the skin is usually white or bluish-pink in color; the chest is prominent and the mammary glands protrude in both sexes.

Time of Birth. The expected time of birth is roughly calculated as 266 days after fertil-

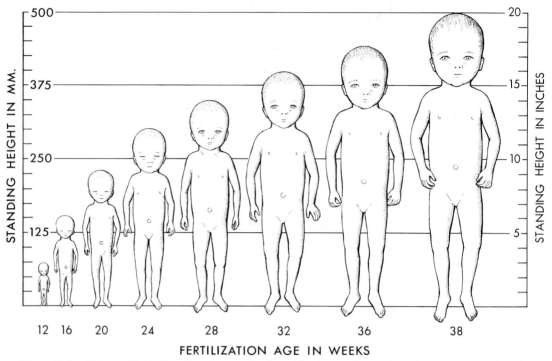

Figure 7–4. Diagram illustrating the changes in size of the human fetus when drawn to scale. (Based on Scammon and Calkins, 1929.)

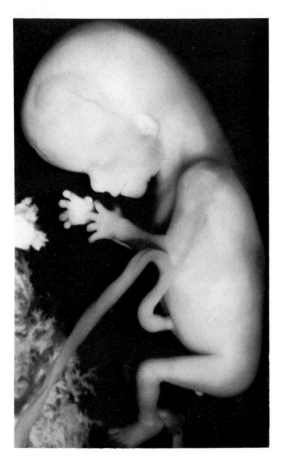

Figure 7–5. Photograph of an 11-week fetus exposed by removal from the chorionic and amniotic sacs (×1.5). Note the relatively large head and that the intestine is no longer in the umbilical cord.

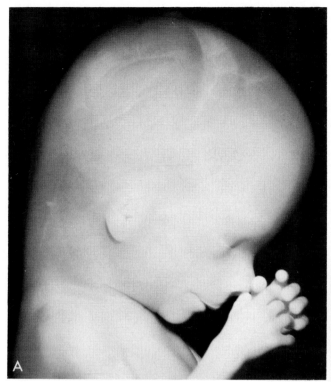

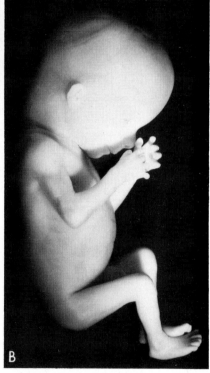

Figure 7–6. Photographs of a 13-week fetus. *A,* Enlarged photograph of the head and shoulders (×2). *B, Actual size.*

ization, or 280 days from the onset of the last menstrual period (Table 7–1). Most fetuses are born within 10 to 15 days of this time, but occasionally birth does not occur until 276 to 286 days after fertilization. A common way of setting the expected date of delivery is to count back three calendar months from the first day of the last menstrual period and then add a year and one week.

FACTORS INFLUENCING FETAL GROWTH

Glucose, Insulin and Amino Acids. Glucose is the primary source of energy for fetal metabolism and growth, but amino acids are also required. These substances are derived from the mother via the placenta (see Chapter 8). Insulin is regarded as a primary growth-regulating hormone for

(Text continued on page 66.)

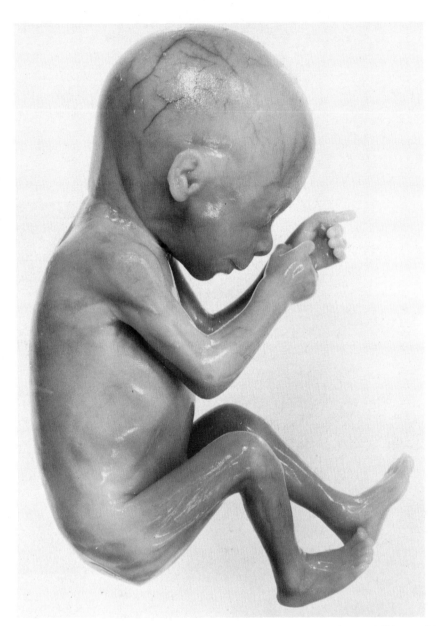

Figure 7–7. Photograph of a 17-week fetus. *Actual size.* Vernix caseosa is not visible on this museum specimen.

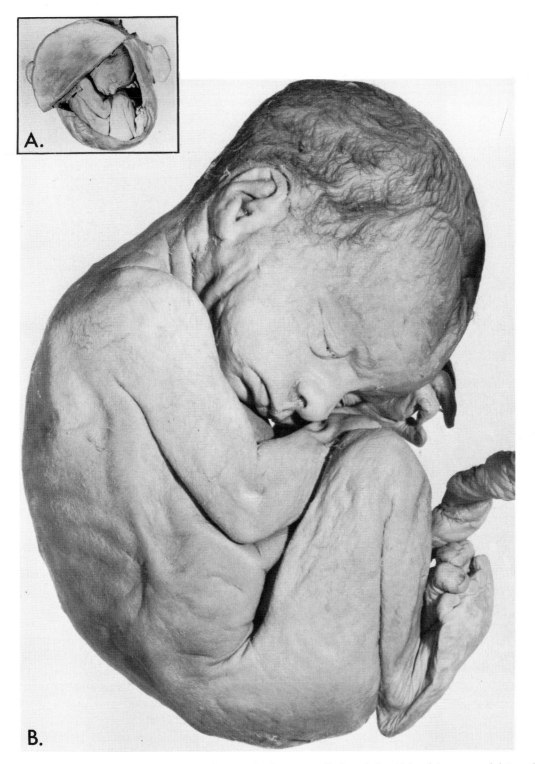

Figure 7–8. Photographs of a 25-week fetus. *A,* In the uterus. *B, Actual size.* Living fetuses are pink to red in color.

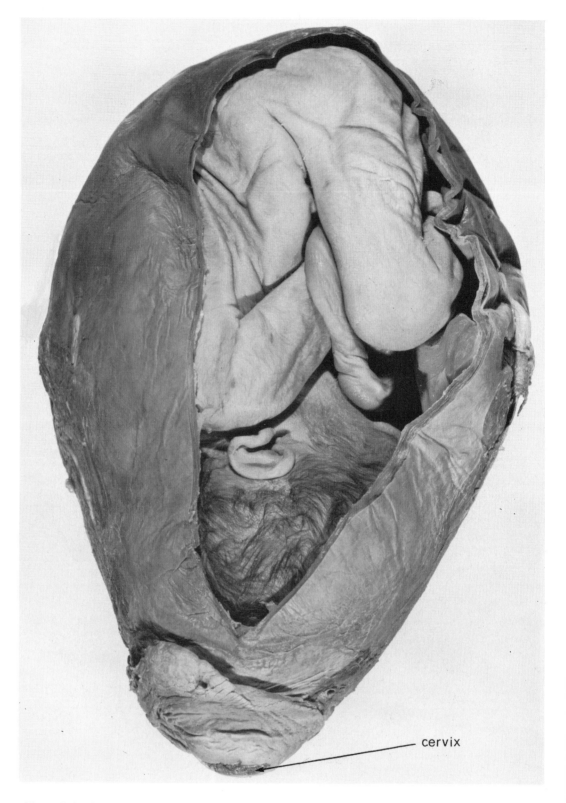

cervix

Figure 7-9. Photograph of a 29-week fetus in the uterus. *Actual size.* Part of the wall of the uterus has been cut away to expose the fetus.

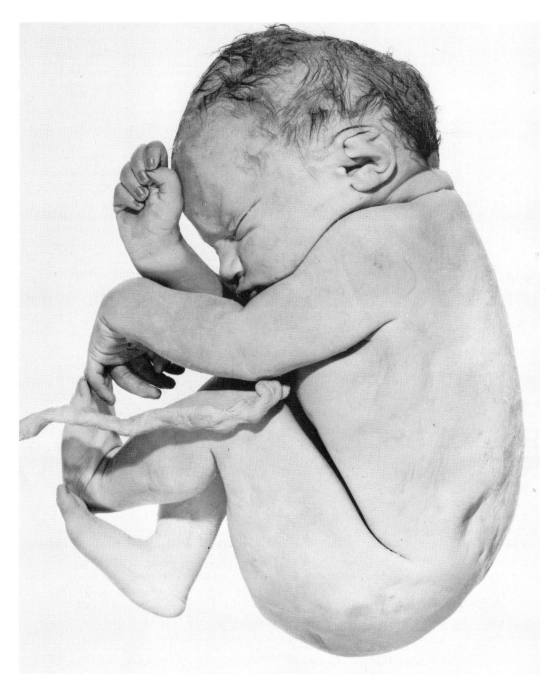

Figure 7–10. Photograph of a 36-week fetus. *Half actual size.*

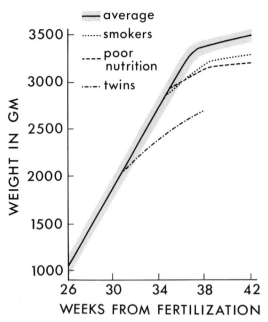

Figure 7–11. Graph showing the rate of fetal growth during the last trimester. (Adapted from Gruenwald, 1966.) Average refers to babies born in the United States. After 36 weeks the growth rate deviates from the straight line. The decline, particularly after full term (38 weeks), probably reflects inadequate fetal nutrition caused by placental changes. Note the adverse effect on fetal weight created by mothers who smoke heavily or eat a poor-quality diet.

the fetus. The insulin required for the metabolism of glucose is secreted by the fetal pancreas. No significant quantities of maternal insulin reach the fetus. Infants of diabetic mothers tend to be larger than normal presumably because of the recurring episodes of hyperglycemia and subsequent hypersecretion of fetal insulin.

Maternal Malnutrition. Severe maternal malnutrition resulting from a poor-quality diet is known to cause reduced fetal growth (Fig. 7–11). Poor nutrition and faulty food habits are common and they are not restricted to mothers belonging to poverty groups.

Smoking. The growth rate of fetuses of mothers who smoke heavily is less than normal during the last six to eight weeks of pregnancy (Fig. 7–11). The effect is greater on fetuses whose mothers also eat a poor-quality diet.

Multiple Pregnancy. Individuals of twins, triplets and other multiple births usually weigh considerably less than infants resulting from a single pregnancy. It is evident

that the total requirements of twins, triplets and so forth exceed the nutritional supply available from the placenta during the third trimester (Fig. 7–11).

Impaired Uteroplacental Blood Flow. Maternal placental circulation may be reduced by a variety of conditions which decrease uterine blood flow (e.g., severe hypotension and renal disease). Chronic reduction of uterine blood flow can cause fetal starvation and result in fetal growth retardation.

Placental Insufficiency. Placental defects can also cause intrauterine fetal growth retardation. These placental changes reduce the total surface area available for exchange of nutrients between the fetal and maternal blood streams (Chapter 8).

Genetic Factors and Chromosomal Aberrations. It is well established that genetic factors can lead to retarded fetal growth. In recent years structural and numerical chromosomal aberrations (Chapter 9) have also been associated with cases of retarded fetal growth.

PERINATOLOGY

Perinatology is the branch of medicine which is primarily concerned with the health of the fetus and newborn infant, generally covering the period from about 26 weeks after fertilization to about four weeks after birth. Several techniques are now available for assessing the status of the human fetus before birth.

Amniocentesis. Amniotic fluid is sampled by inserting a hollow needle through the mother's abdominal wall into the amniotic cavity. A syringe is then attached and amniotic fluid withdrawn. Amniotic fluid examination by this method is now a major tool in assessing the degree of erythroblastosis fetalis (also called hemolytic disease of the fetus and newborn). This condition results from destruction of fetal red blood cells by maternal antibodies (see Chapter 8).

Sex Chromatin Patterns. Fetal sex can be diagnosed by noting the presence or absence of sex chromatin in cells recovered from amniotic fluid (Fig. 7–12). Knowledge of fetal sex can be useful in diagnosing the presence of severe sex-linked hereditary diseases such as hemophilia or muscular dystrophy. *These tests are not done merely to diagnose fetal sex for curious parents.*

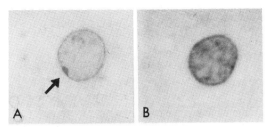

Figure 7–12. Nuclei of cells in amniotic fluid obtained by amniocentesis. *A*, Chromatin positive nucleus indicating the presence of a female fetus; the sex chromatin is indicated by an arrow. *B*, Chromatin negative nucleus indicating the presence of a male fetus. No sex chromatin is visible. Cresyl echt violet stain. ×1000. (From Riis, M., and Fuchs, F.: Sex chromatin and antenatal sex diagnosis. *In* K. L. Moore [Ed.]: *The Sex Chromatin*, 1966. Courtesy of the W. B. Saunders Co.)

Cell Cultures. Fetal sex can also be determined by studying the sex chromosomes of cultured amniotic cells. These studies are more commonly done when an autosomal abnormality is suspected, such as occurs in Down's syndrome (discussed in Chapter 9). Inborn errors of metabolism and enzyme deficiencies in fetuses can also be detected by studying cell cultures. Cell cultures permit prenatal diagnosis of severe diseases for which there is no effective treatment and afford the opportunity to interrupt the pregnancy.

Intrauterine Transfusion. Some fetuses with erythroblastosis fetalis can be saved by giving them intrauterine blood transfusions. The blood is injected through a needle inserted into the fetal peritoneal cavity. Over a period of five to six days, most of the cells pass into the fetal circulation via the lymphatics of the diaphragm.

Fetal Blood Samples. Using an instrument called an endoscope inserted into the cervix, blood samples can be obtained from a fetus, usually from the scalp.

SUMMARY

The fetal period begins about eight weeks after fertilization and ends at birth. It is primarily characterized by rapid body growth and maturation of organ systems. An obvious change is the relative slowing of head growth compared with that of the rest of the body. Lanugo and head hair appear, and the skin is coated with vernix caseosa by the beginning of the twentieth week. The eyelids are fused during much of the fetal period but reopen at about 26 weeks. Until this time the fetus is incapable of extrauterine existence, mainly because of the immaturity of the respiratory system. Fat usually develops rapidly during the last six to eight weeks, making the fetus smooth and plump. This terminal period is devoted mainly to building up of tissues and preparation of systems involved in the transition from intrauterine to extrauterine environments.

Changes occurring during the fetal period are not so dramatic as those in the embryonic period, but they are very important. The fetus is far less vulnerable to the teratogenic or deforming effects of drugs, viruses and radiation, but these agents may interfere with normal functional development, especially of the brain. Various techniques are available for assessing the status of the fetus and for diagnosing certain diseases and developmental abnormalities before birth.

8

THE PLACENTA
AND FETAL
MEMBRANES

The *chorion*, the *amnion*, the *yolk sac* and the *allantois* constitute the embryonic[1] or fetal membranes. These nutritive and protective membranes develop from the zygote but do not form embryonic structures, except for portions of the yolk sac and allantois. Before birth, the placenta and fetal membranes perform the following functions and activities: *protection, nutrition, respiration* and *excretion.* At birth, the placenta and fetal membranes are separated from the fetus and expelled from the uterus as the afterbirth.

THE DECIDUA

The term decidua[2] is applied to the functional layer of the gravid or pregnant endometrium, indicating that it is shed at parturition. Three regions of decidua are designated according to their relation to the implantation site (Fig. 8–1): (1) the part underlying the conceptus and forming the maternal component of the placenta is the *decidua basalis;* (2) the superficial portion overlying the conceptus is the *decidua capsularis;* and (3) all the remaining uterine mucosa is the *decidua parietalis.* As the con-

ceptus enlarges, the decidua capsularis bulges into the uterine cavity and eventually fuses with the decidua parietalis, thus obliterating the uterine cavity (Fig. 8–1*F*). By about 22 weeks, the decidua capsularis degenerates and disappears.

DEVELOPMENT OF THE PLACENTA

The rapid proliferation of the trophoblast and development of the chorionic sac were described in Chapters 4 and 5. By the fourth week, the essential arrangements necessary for physiological exchanges between the mother and embryo are established. Villi cover the entire surface of the chorionic sac until about the eighth week (Figs. 8–1*C* and 8–2*A*). As the sac grows, the villi associated with the decidua capsularis become compressed and their blood supply reduced. Subsequently, these villi degenerate, producing a bare area known as the *smooth chorion* (Figs. 8–1*D* and 8–2*B*). As this occurs, the villi associated with the decidua basalis rapidly increase in number, branch profusely and enlarge. This portion of the chorionic sac, known as the *villous chorion*, forms the fetal component of the placenta (Fig. 8–1*F*). The final shape of the placenta is determined by the form of the persistent area of villi; usually this is circular, giving the placenta a discoid shape (Fig. 8–3). As the villi erode the decidua basalis, they leave

---

[1] Sometimes called extraembryonic membranes to indicate that they are not part of the embryo.

[2] From Latin *deciduus,* "a falling-off," as of the leaves of deciduous trees in the autumn.

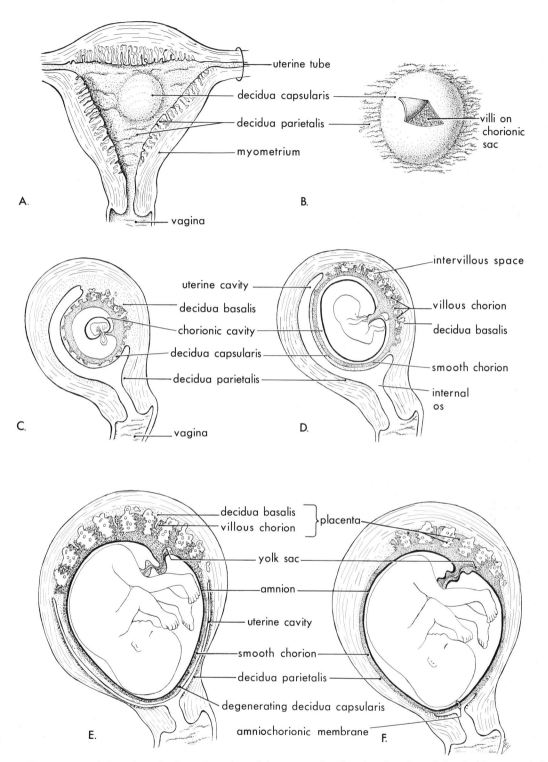

A. uterine tube

decidua capsularis

decidua parietalis

myometrium

vagina

B. villi on chorionic sac

intervillous space

uterine cavity

decidua basalis

chorionic cavity

decidua capsularis

decidua parietalis

villous chorion

decidua basalis

smooth chorion

internal os

C. vagina

D.

decidua basalis

villous chorion } placenta

yolk sac

amnion

uterine cavity

smooth chorion

decidua parietalis

degenerating decidua capsularis

amniochorionic membrane

E.

F.

Figure 8–1. *A,* Drawing of a frontal section of the uterus showing the elevation of the decidua capsularis caused by the expanding chorionic sac of an implanted four-week embryo. *B,* Enlarged drawing of the implantation site; the chorionic villi have been exposed by cutting an opening in the decidua capsularis. *C* to *F,* Drawings of sagittal sections of the gravid uterus from the fourth to twenty-second weeks, showing the changing relations of the fetal membranes to the decidua. In *F,* the amnion and chorion are fused with each other and the decidua parietalis, thus obliterating the uterine cavity. Note that the villi persist only where the chorion is associated with the decidua basalis, and that initially the placenta is larger than the fetus. During the last half of pregnancy the fetus grows faster than the placenta.

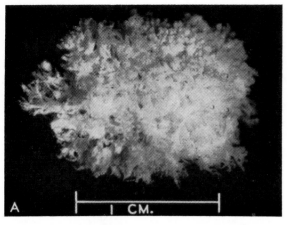

smooth
chorion

villous
chorion

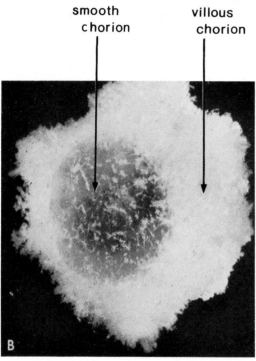

Figure 8–2. Photographs of human chorionic sacs. *A,* 21 days. The entire sac is covered with tertiary chorionic villi (×4). *B,* Eight weeks. *Actual size.* Note that some villi have degenerated, leaving the smooth chorion. The remaining villous chorion forms the fetal contribution to the placenta. (From Potter, E. L.: *Pathology of the Fetus and Infant.* 2nd Ed., 1961. Courtesy of Year Book Medical Publishers, Inc.)

several wedge-shaped areas of decidual tissue called placental septa (Fig. 8–5). These septa divide the fetal part of the placenta into 15 to 30 irregular areas called *cotyledons* (Fig. 8–10*A*). The fetal portion of the placenta (or villous chorion) is anchored to the maternal portion of the placenta (or decidua basalis) by *anchoring villi* (Fig. 8–5).

The Intervillous Space. The blood-filled intervillous spaces (Figs. 8–1*D* and 8–4) are derived mainly from the lacunae which developed in the syncytiotrophoblast during the second week. During subsequent erosion by the trophoblast, these spaces enlarge at the expense of the decidua basalis. Collec-

tively, the spaces form a large blood sinus, the *intervillous space,* which is bounded by the chorionic plate and decidua basalis (Figs. 8–4 and 8–5). The marginal portion of the intervillous space is often called the *marginal sinus* or lake (Fig. 8–5). The intervillous space is drained by endometrial veins which open on the surface of the decidua basalis (Fig. 8–5).

PLACENTAL CIRCULATION

The placenta provides a large area where materials may be exchanged across the pla-

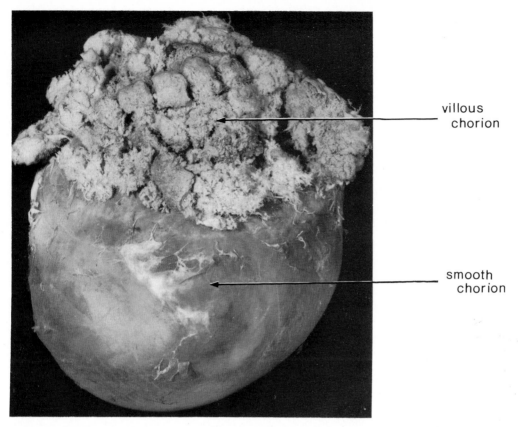

villous
chorion

smooth
chorion

Figure 8–3. Photograph of a human chorionic sac containing a 13-week fetus showing the smooth and villous areas of the chorion. *Actual size.*

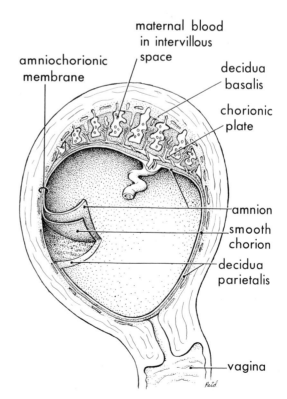

maternal blood
in intervillous
space

amniochorionic
membrane

decidua
basalis

chorionic
plate

amnion

smooth
chorion

decidua
parietalis

vagina

Figure 8–4. Drawing of a sagittal section of the gravid uterus at 22 weeks showing the relations of the fetal membranes to each other and to the decidua. The fetus has been removed, and the amnion and smooth chorion have been cut and reflected.

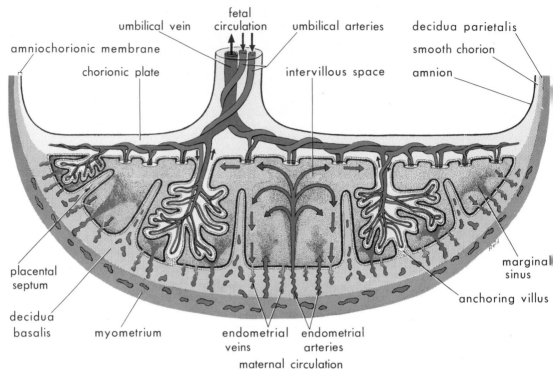

Figure 8–5. Schematic drawing of a section through a mature placenta. Maternal blood is driven into the intervillous space in funnel-shaped spurts, and exchanges occur with the fetal blood as the maternal blood flows around the villi. The inflowing arterial blood pushes venous blood out into the endometrial veins, which are scattered over the entire surface of the decidua basalis. Note that the umbilical arteries carry deoxygenated fetal blood (shown in blue) to the placenta and that the umbilical vein carries oxygenated blood (shown in red) to the fetus. (Based on Ramsey, 1965.)

cental membrane interposed between the fetal and maternal circulations (Fig. 8–7). From the maternal blood the fetal blood acquires nutrients and oxygen. Waste products formed within the embryo are carried to the placenta and transferred to the maternal blood. Within the placenta, the maternal and fetal blood streams flow close to each other, but are not continuous.

The Placental Membrane. This membrane consists of the fetal tissues separating the maternal and fetal blood. Until about 20 weeks, it consists of four layers (Fig. 8–6B): (1) the syncytiotrophoblast, (2) the cytotrophoblast, (3) the connective tissue core of the villus, and (4) the endothelium of the fetal capillary. As pregnancy advances, the placental membrane becomes progressively thinner and many capillaries come to lie very close to the syncytiotrophoblast (Fig. 8–6C). At some sites the syncytiotrophoblastic nuclei form nuclear aggregations or *syncytial*

knots. Toward the end of pregnancy, *fibrinoid material* forms on the surfaces of villi; it consists of fibrin and other substances. These changes result mainly from aging.

Fetal Placental Circulation. Deoxygenated blood leaves the fetus and passes in the umbilical arteries to the placenta (Fig. 8–5). The blood vessels form an extensive *arterio-capillary-venous system* within the villus (Fig. 8–6A), bringing the fetal blood very close to the maternal blood. The oxygenated fetal blood passes into thin-walled veins which converge to form the umbilical vein. This large vessel carries the oxygenated blood to the fetus (Fig. 8–5).

Maternal Placental Circulation. Blood in the intervillous space is temporarily outside the maternal circulatory system; it enters the intervillous space through 80 to 100 *spiral endometrial arteries* (Fig. 8–5). The blood is propelled in jet-like streams by the

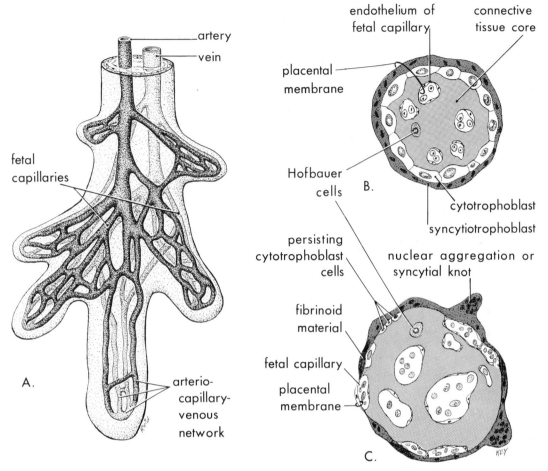

Figure 8–6. *A,* Drawing of a tertiary chorionic villus showing the course of fetal blood vessels. *B* and *C,* Drawings of sections through a chorionic villus at 10 weeks and at full term, respectively. The Hofbauer cells have the general properties of macrophages, which are cells that are active in the defense of the body against microorganisms.

maternal blood pressure and spurts toward the chorionic plate or "roof" of the placenta. The blood slowly flows around and over the surface of the villi, allowing an exchange of metabolic and gaseous products with the fetal blood. The maternal blood eventually reaches the floor of the intervillous space, where it enters the endometrial veins.

PLACENTAL FUNCTIONS

The placenta has three main activities: (1) metabolism, (2) transfer, and (3) endocrine secretion; all are essential for maintaining pregnancy and promoting normal embryonic development. The placenta synthesizes glycogen, cholesterol and fatty acids.

Gases. Oxygen, carbon dioxide and carbon monoxide cross the placental membrane by simple diffusion (Fig. 8–7). Interruption of oxygen transport for even a few minutes will endanger fetal survival.

Nutrients. Water is rapidly and freely exchanged between mother and fetus. There is little or no transfer of maternal cholesterol, triglycerides or phospholipids. There is transport of free fatty acids, but the amount transferred is probably relatively small. Vitamins cross the placenta and are essential for normal development. Water-soluble vitamins cross the placental membrane more quickly than fat-soluble ones. Glucose is quickly transferred.

Hormones. Protein hormones do not reach the fetus in significant amounts, ex-

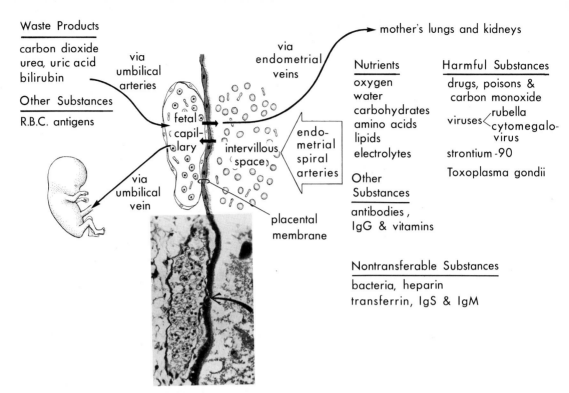

Figure 8–7. Diagrammatic illustration of placental transfer. The inset photomicrograph is from Javert, C. T.: *Spontaneous and Habitual Abortion.* 1957. Courtesy of The Blakiston Division, McGraw-Hill Book Co.

cept for a slow transfer of thyroxine and triiodothyronine. Unconjugated steroid hormones pass the placental membrane rather freely, unless they are firmly bound to proteins. Testosterone and certain synthetic progestins cross the placenta and may cause external masculinization of female fetuses (see Chapter 9).

Electrolytes. These are freely exchanged across the placenta in significant quantities, each at its own rate. It is important to realize that when a mother receives intravenous fluids, they also pass to the fetus and affect its water and electrolyte status.

Antibodies. Some passive immunity is conferred upon the fetus by transplacental transfer of maternal antibodies. The alpha and beta globulins reach the fetus in very small quantities, but many of the gamma globulins, notably the IgG (7S) class, are readily transported to the fetus. Maternal antibodies confer immunity on the fetus to such diseases as diphtheria, smallpox and measles, but no immunity is acquired to pertussis (whooping cough) or chickenpox.

Although the placental membrane separates the maternal and fetal circulations,

small amounts of blood may pass from the fetus to the mother. If the fetus is Rh positive and the mother Rh negative, the fetal red blood cell antigens elicit an antibody response in the mother. The maternal antibodies then cross the placenta and enter the fetal circulation, causing a breakdown of red blood cells. Some fetuses with this condition, known as *erythroblastosis fetalis* or hemolytic disease of the fetus, fail to make a satisfactory intrauterine adjustment and die unless delivered early or given intrauterine blood transfusions (discussed in Chapter 7).

Wastes. The major waste product, carbon dioxide, diffuses across the placenta even more rapidly than oxygen. Urea and uric acid pass the placental membrane by simple diffusion.

Drugs. Most drugs cross the placenta freely; some cause congenital malformations (see Chapter 9). Fetal drug addiction may occur following maternal use of drugs such as heroin. Except for the muscle relaxants, such as succinylcholine and curare, most agents used for the management of labor readily cross the placenta. These drugs may cause respiratory depression of the newborn infant. All sedatives and analgesics affect the fetus to some degree.

Infectious agents. Rubella and coxsackie viruses and those associated with variola, varicella, measles, encephalitis and poliomyelitis may pass through the placental membrane and cause fetal infection. In some cases (e. g., rubella virus), congenital malformations may be produced (Chapter 9).

Endocrine secretion

The *syncytiotrophoblast* synthesizes the following hormones:

Protein hormones. The three well-documented protein products of the placenta are :(1) *human chorionic gonadotropin* (HCG), (2) human chorionic somatomammotropin (HCS) or human placental lactogen (HPL), and (3) *thyrotropin.*

Steroid hormones. Estrogens and progesterones are the only steroid hormones known to be secreted by the placenta.

FETAL AND UTERINE GROWTH

The uterus normally lies entirely in the pelvis (Fig. 8–8*A*). During pregnancy the uterus expands as the fetus grows, and rises out of the pelvic cavity to the level of the mother's umbilicus (navel) by about 16 weeks (Fig. 8–8*B*). By 32 weeks, the uterus in the pregnant female occupies a large part of the abdomino-pelvic cavity (Fig. 8–8*C*).

PARTURITION OR LABOR

The processes of birth are referred to as parturition or labor (Fig. 8–9). The onset of labor is caused mainly by hormonal influences. Although occurring in a continuous sequence, labor is divided into three stages for convenience of description. The *first stage* is the dilatation stage. The amnion and chorion are forced into the cervical canal by contractions of the uterus (Fig. 8–9*A*). The cervix dilates slowly, and when it is fully dilated, or even before, the amniotic and chorionic sacs rupture, allowing the fluid to escape. During the *second stage,* the contractions of the uterus become stronger and are aided by voluntary contractions of the maternal abdominal muscles. The baby is forced through the cervical canal and the vagina (Fig. 8–9*B* to *E*). The *third stage* is the interval from birth to the expulsion of the placenta and membranes, which are now referred to as the "afterbirth."

THE FULL-TERM PLACENTA AND UMBILICAL CORD

The placenta (from Greek *plakuos,* "a flat cake") commonly has the form of a flat

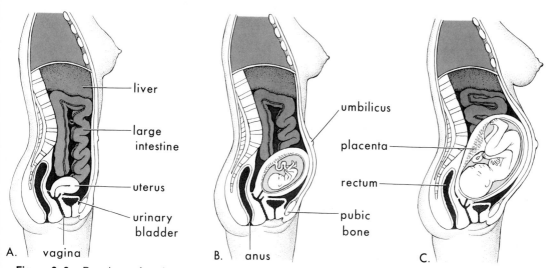

Figure 8–8. Drawings of sagittal sections of a female. *A,* Not pregnant. *B,* 16 weeks pregnant. *C,* 32 weeks pregnant. Note that as the fetus enlarges, the uterus increases in size and its upper part rises out of the pelvic cavity. The mother's intestines are displaced by the growth of the fetus and uterus.

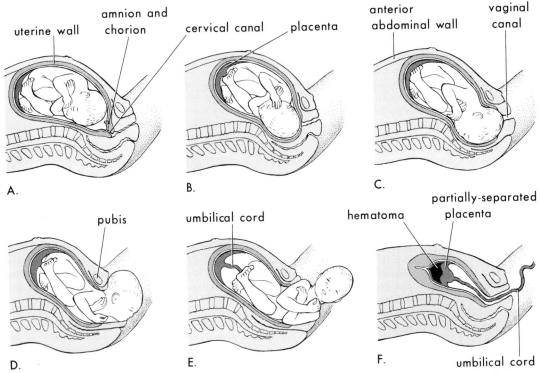

Figure 8–9. Drawings illustrating the processes of birth. *A* and *B,* The cervix is dilating during the first stage of labor as the result of the amnion and chorion being forced into the cervical canal. *C* to *E,* The fetus passes through the cervix and vagina during the second stage of labor. *F,* As the uterus contracts during the third stage of labor, the placenta folds up and pulls away from the uterine wall. Separation of the placenta results in bleeding, forming a large hematoma. Later the placenta and its associated membranes are expelled from the uterus (not shown) by further uterine contractions.

circular or oval disc (Fig. 8–10) with a diameter of 15 to 20 cm and a thickness of 2 to 3 cm. The placenta weighs 500 to 600 gm, usually about one-sixth the weight of the fetus. The margins of the placenta are continuous with the ruptured amniotic and chorionic sacs (Figs. 8–5 and 8–10*A* and *C*).

Maternal Surface (Fig. 8–9*A*). The characteristic cobblestone appearance of this surface is caused by the 15 to 30 cotyledons. The surface of the cotyledons is usually covered by thin, grayish shreds of decidua basalis. Most of the decidua, however, is temporarily retained in the uterus and shed with subsequent uterine bleeding.

Fetal Surface (Fig. 8–10*B*). The umbilical cord attaches to this surface, and its amniotic covering is continuous with the amnion adherent to this surface of the placenta. The vessels radiating from the umbilical cord are clearly visible through the smooth transparent amnion. Several variations in placental shape occur, e. g., accessory placenta (Fig. 8–11), bidiscoid placenta and diffuse placenta.

The Umbilical Cord

The attachment of the umbilical cord is usually near the center of the placenta. The cord is usually 1 to 2 cm in diameter and 50 to 55 cm in length. The umbilical cord usually contains two arteries and one vein. These vessels are surrounded by mucoid connective tissue, often called Wharton's jelly (Fig. 8–12*A*). Because the umbilical vein is longer than the arteries and the vessels are longer than the cord, twisting and bending of the vessels is common. The vessels frequently form loops, producing so-called *false knots* which are of no significance. True knots in the cord may be hazardous to the fetus (Fig. 8–13). Simple looping of the cord around the fetus occasionally occurs (Fig. 8–15). In about one-fifth of all deliveries, the cord is looped once around the neck. In up to one per cent of newborns, only one umbilical artery is present (Fig. 8–12*B*), a condition often associated with fetal abnormalities, particularly of the cardiovascular system.

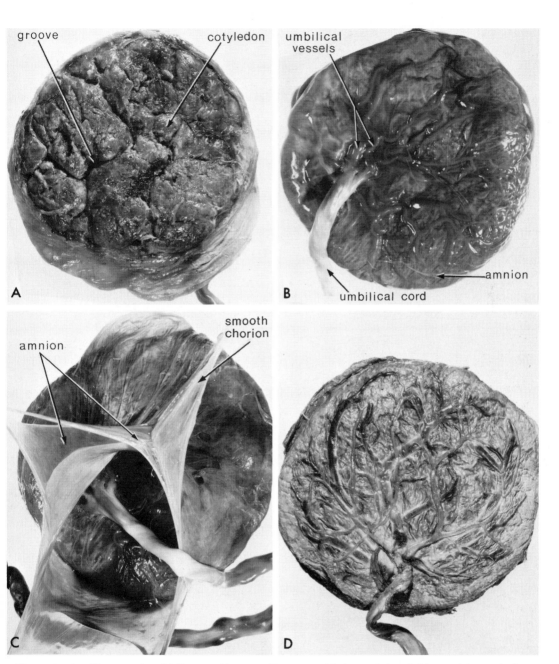

Figure 8–10.   Photographs of full term placentas. *About one-third actual size. A,* Maternal (or uterine) surface, showing cotyledons and grooves. *B,* Fetal (or amniotic) surface, showing the blood vessels running under the amnion and converging to form the umbilical vessels at the attachment of the umbilical cord. *C,* The amnion and smooth chorion are arranged to show that they are (1) fused and (2) continuous with the margins of the placenta. *D,* Placenta with a marginal attachment of the cord, often called a battledore placenta because of its resemblance to the bat used in the medieval game of battledore and shuttlecock.

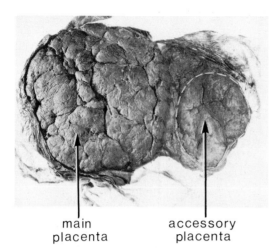

Figure 8–11. Photograph of the maternal surface of a full term placenta with an associated accessory placenta. *About one-quarter actual size.*

main placenta   accessory placenta

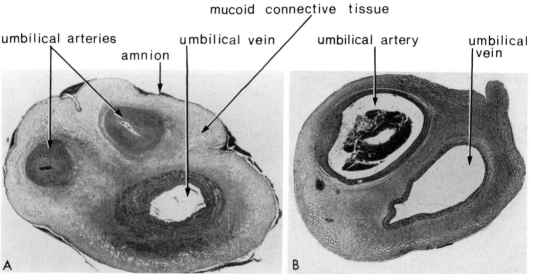

mucoid connective tissue

umbilical arteries   amnion   umbilical vein   umbilical artery   umbilical vein

A   B

Figure 8–12. Transverse sections through full term umbilical cords. *A,* Normal. *B,* Abnormal, showing only one artery. (×3.) (From Javert, C. T.: *Spontaneous and Habitual Abortion.* 1957. Courtesy of The Blakiston Division, McGraw-Hill Book Co.)

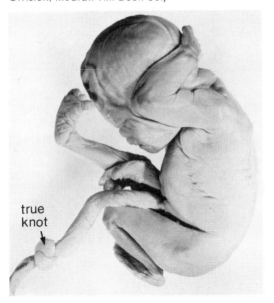

true knot

Figure 8–13. Photograph of a 20-week fetus with a true knot (arrow) in the umbilical cord. *Half actual size.* The diameter of the cord is greater in the portion closest to the fetus, indicating that there was an obstruction of blood flow in the umbilical arteries.

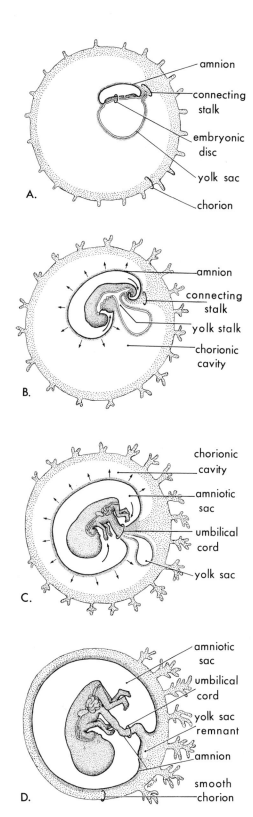

THE AMNION AND AMNIOTIC FLUID

Formation of the amniotic cavity and early development of the amnion are described in Chapter 4. Because the amnion is attached to the margins of the embryonic disc (Fig. 8–14*A*), its junction with the embryo becomes located on the ventral surface as a result of folding of the embryo (see Chapter 6). As the amniotic sac enlarges, it gradually sheaths the umbilical cord, forming its epithelial covering (Fig. 8–14*C* and *D*).

Origin of Amniotic Fluid. Initially, most fluid is derived from the maternal blood. Later, the fetus also makes a contribution by excreting urine into the amniotic fluid. Amniotic fluid is normally swallowed by the fetus and subsequently absorbed by the gastrointestinal tract. In fetal conditions such as renal agenesis (absence of kidneys) or urethral obstruction, the volume of amniotic fluid may be abnormally small (oligohydramnios). An excess of amniotic fluid (polyhydramnios) may occur when the fetus does not drink the usual amount of fluid. This condition is often associated with malformations of the central nervous system, e.g., anencephaly and hydrocephalus (see Chapter 17). In other malformations, such as esophageal or duodenal atresia (see Chapter 13), amniotic fluid accumulates because it is unable to pass to the intestine for absorption.

Significance of Amniotic Fluid. The embryo, suspended by the umbilical cord, floats freely in amniotic fluid. This buoyant medium (1) permits symmetrical growth and development of the embryo; (2) prevents adherence of the amnion to the embryo; (3) cushions the embryo against jolts by distributing impacts the mother may receive; (4) helps to control the embryo's body temperature by maintaining a relatively constant temperature; and (5) enables the fetus to move freely, thus aiding musculoskeletal development.

THE YOLK SAC

Early development of the yolk sac is described in Chapters 4 and 5. By nine weeks, the yolk sac has shrunk to a pear-shaped remnant, about 5 mm in diameter, which is connected to the midgut by the narrow yolk stalk (Fig. 8–14*C*). Although the human

Figure 8–14. Drawings illustrating how the amnion becomes the outer covering of the umbilical cord and how the yolk sac is partially incorporated into the embryo as the primitive gut. *A*, Three weeks. *B*, Four weeks. *C*, 10 weeks. *D*, 20 weeks.

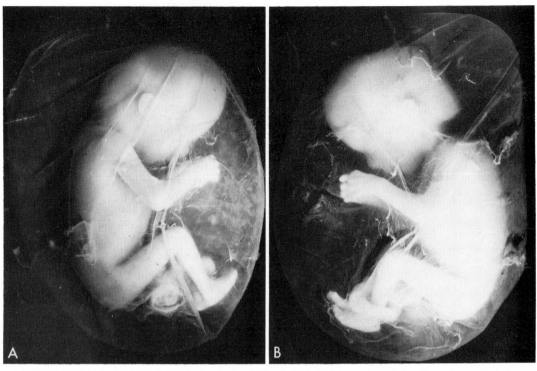

Figure 8–15. Photographs of a 12-week fetus within the amniotic sac. *Actual size.* Note the umbilical cord looped around the left foot of the fetus.

yolk sac is nonfunctional as far as yolk storage is concerned, its development is essential for several reasons. (1) It appears to have a role in the transfer of nutrients to the embryo during the second and third weeks while the uteroplacental circulation is being established. (2) Blood develops on the walls of the yolk sac beginning in the third week and continues to form here until hemopoietic activity begins in the liver during the sixth week. (3) During the fourth week, the dorsal part of the yolk sac is incorporated into the embryo as the primitive gut; this gives rise to the epithelium of the trachea, bronchi and lungs, and of the digestive tract. (4) Primordial germ cells appear in the wall of the yolk sac early in the third week and subsequently migrate to the developing sex glands or gonads, where they become the primitive germ cells (spermatogonia or oogonia — see Chapter 14).

Fate of the Yolk Sac. The yolk sac shrinks as pregnancy advances and eventually becomes very small. The yolk stalk usually detaches from the gut by the end of the fifth week. In about two per cent of adults, the intra-abdominal part of the yolk stalk persists as a diverticulum of the ileum known as *Meckel's diverticulum* (see Chapter 13).

THE ALLANTOIS

The early development of the allantois is described in Chapter 5. Although the allantois does not function in human embryos, it is important for two reasons: (1) blood formation occurs on its walls during the first two months; and (2) its blood vessels become the umbilical vein and arteries (Fig. 8–16*A* and *B*).

Fate of the Allantois. During the second month, the extraembryonic portion of the allantois degenerates. The intraembryonic portion of the allantois runs from the umbilicus to the urinary bladder with which it is continuous (Fig. 8–16*B*). As the bladder enlarges, the allantois involutes to form a thick tube called the *urachus.* After birth, the urachus becomes a fibrous cord called the median umbilical ligament.

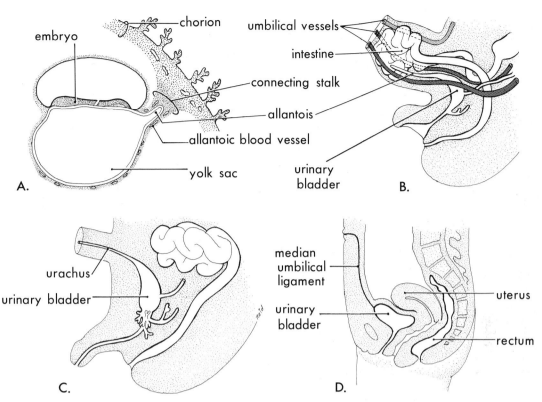

Figure 8–16. Drawings illustrating the development and usual fate of the allantois. *A*, Three weeks. *B*, Nine weeks. *C*, Three months. *D*, Adult.

MULTIPLE PREGNANCY

Twins

Twins may originate from two zygotes (Fig. 8–17), in which case they are dizygotic, nonidentical or fraternal, or from one zygote (Fig. 8–18), i. e., monozygotic or identical. Twins occur about once in 80 to 90 pregnancies; about two-thirds of the total number are dizygotic twins. In addition, the rate of monozygotic twinning shows little variation with the mother's age, whereas dizygotic twinning increases with maternal age.

There is a tendency for dizygotic, but not monozygotic, twins to repeat in families. It has also been found that if the firstborn are twins, a repetition of twinning or some other form of multiple birth is about five times more likely to occur at the next pregnancy than it is in the general population.

Dizygotic Twins. Because they result from the fertilization of two ova by different sperms, the twins may be of the same sex or of different sexes. For the same reason, they are no more alike genetically than brothers or sisters born at different times. Dizygotic twins always have two amnions and two chorions, but the chorions and placentas may be fused (Fig. 8–17).

Monozygotic Twins. Because they result from the fertilization of one ovum (Fig. 8–18), the twins are (1) of the same sex, (2) genetically identical, and (3) very similar in physical appearance. Physical differences between identical twins are caused by environmental factors, e.g., anastomosis of placental vessels (Fig. 8–19). Monozygotic twinning usually begins around the end of the first week and results from division of the inner cell mass into two embryonic primordia. Subsequently, two identical embryos, each in its own amniotic sac, develop within one chorionic sac. The twins have a common placenta and often some placental vessels join (Fig. 8–18).

Very rarely, later division of embryonic cells results in monozygotic twins which are in one amniotic and one chorionic sac (Fig. 8–20*A*). Such twins are rarely delivered alive

(*Text continued on page 86.*)

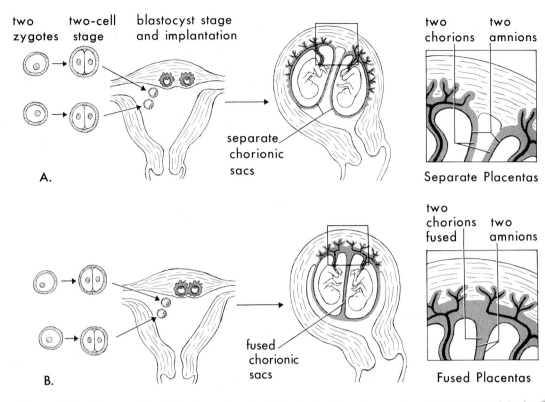

Figure 8–17. Diagrams illustrating how dizygotic twins develop from two zygotes. The relations of the fetal membranes and placentas are shown for instances in which, *A,* the blastocysts implant separately, and *B,* the blastocysts implant close together. In both cases there are two amnions and two chorions, and the placentas may be separate or fused.

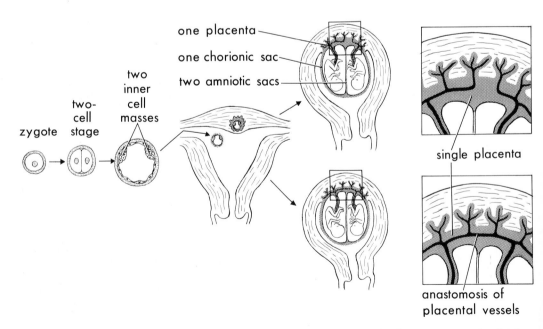

Figure 8–18. Diagrams illustrating how monozygotic twins usually develop from one zygote by division of the inner cell mass. Such twins always have separate amnions, a single chorion and a common placenta.

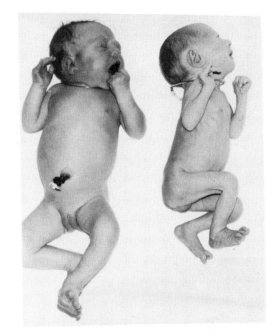

Figure 8-19. Monozygotic (or "identical") twins showing a wide discrepancy in size resulting from an uncompensated arteriovenous anastomosis of placental vessels. Blood was shunted from the smaller twin to the larger twin, producing the so-called fetal transfusion syndrome. (Courtesy of Dr. Harry Medovy, Children's Centre, Winnipeg.)

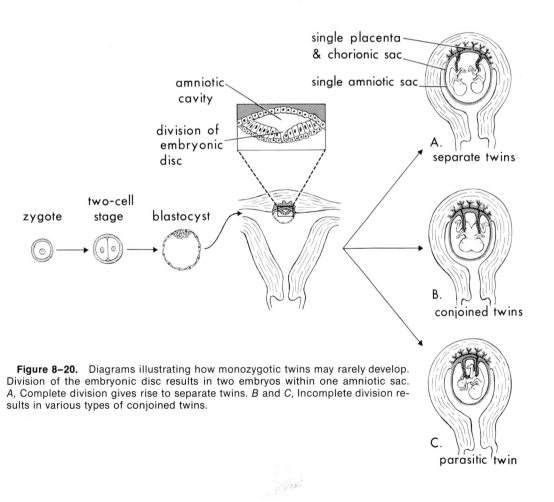

Figure 8-20. Diagrams illustrating how monozygotic twins may rarely develop. Division of the embryonic disc results in two embryos within one amniotic sac. *A,* Complete division gives rise to separate twins. *B* and *C,* Incomplete division results in various types of conjoined twins.

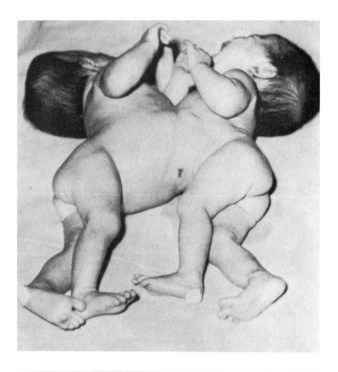

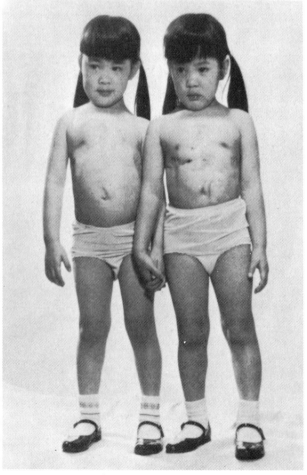

Figure 8–21. *A,* Photograph of newborn conjoined twins showing ventral union (thoracopagus). *B,* The twins about four years after separation. (From de Vries, P. A.: Case history—the San Francisco twins; *In* Bergsma, D. [Ed.]: *Conjoined Twins. Birth Defects. Original Article Series,* Vol. III, No. 1, April, 1967. © The National Foundation, New York.)

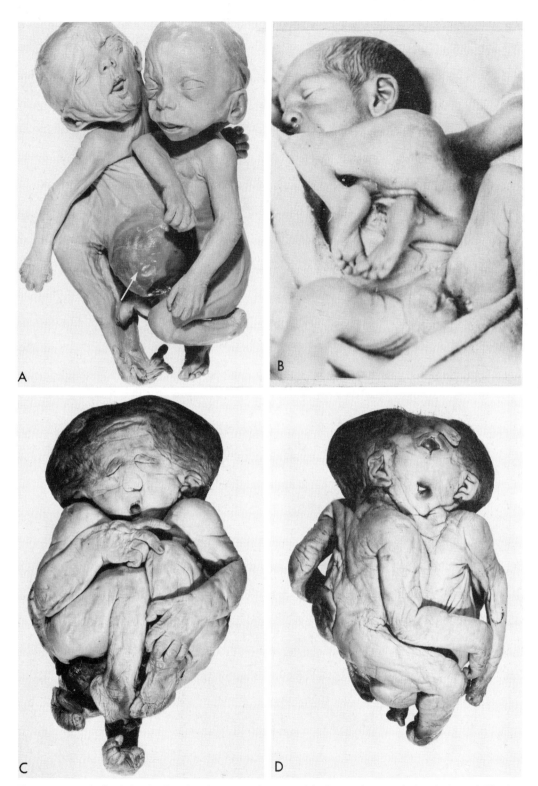

Figure 8–22. *A,* Conjoined twins showing extensive ventral fusion and an omphalocele (arrow). The lower extremities of the left fetus are fused, a condition known as sirenomelus. *B,* Parasitic fetus with fairly well developed legs and pelvis attached to the thorax of an otherwise normal male infant. (Courtesy of Dr. L. A. Sigurdson, Winnipeg.) *C* and *D,* Two views of conjoined twins showing the so-called janiceps abnormality with two faces and fusion of the cranial and thoracic regions (cephalothoracopagus).

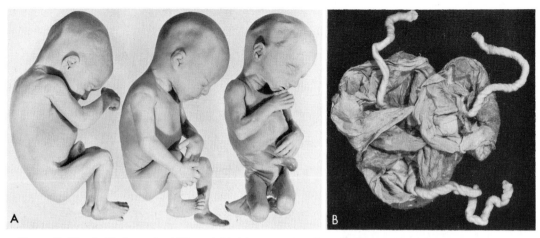

Figure 8–23. *A*, Photograph of 20-week triplets: monozygotic male twins (left) and a single female (right). *B*, Photograph of their fused placentas shows the twin placenta with two amnions (left) and the single placenta (upper right).

because the umbilical cords are frequently entangled so that circulation ceases and one or both fetuses die.

Conjoined Twins. If the embryonic disc does not divide completely, various types of conjoined twins may form (Figs. 8–20*B* and *C*, 8–21 and 8–22). These are named according to the regions that are attached, e.g., "thoracopagus," which indicates that

there is ventral union of the thoracic regions (Fig. 8–21).

Other Multiple Births

Triplets occur once in about 7600 pregnancies and may be derived from (1) one

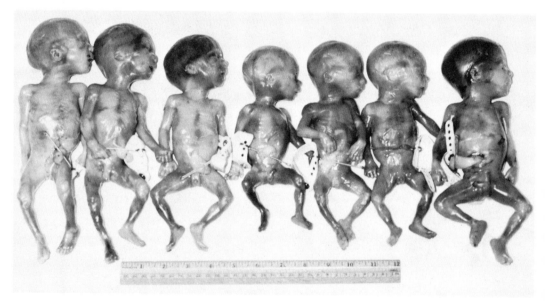

Figure 8–24. Photograph of septuplets, five female and two male, of about 17 weeks. Study of the fetal membranes indicated that they were probably derived from seven ova. (From Turksoy *et al.*: *Obstet. Gynec.* 30:692, 1967.)

zygote and be identical, (2) two zygotes and consist of identical twins and a single infant (Fig. 8–23), or (3) three zygotes and be of the same sex or of different sexes. In the last case, the infants are no more similar than those from three separate pregnancies. Similar possible combinations occur in *quadruplets, quintuplets, sextuplets, septuplets* and so forth. Types of multiple births higher than triplets are normally very rare, but they have occurred more often in recent years following the administration of gonadotropins to women with ovulatory failure (Fig. 8–24).

SUMMARY

In addition to the embryo, the zygote gives rise to the fetal membranes and most of the placenta. The placenta consists of two parts: (1) a fetal portion derived from the *villous chorion*, and (2) a maternal portion formed by the *decidua basalis*. The two parts work together in placental transfer. The fetal circulation is separated from the maternal circulation by a thin layer of fetal tissues known as the *placental membrane*. The principal activities of the placenta are (1) metabolism, (2) transfer, and (3) endocrine secretion.

The fetal membranes and placenta(s) in multiple pregnancy vary considerably depending on the derivation of the embryos and when division of the embryonic cells occurs. The common type of twins is dizygotic, with two amnions, two chorions and two placentas which may or may not be fused. About a third of all twins are derived from one zygote; these commonly have two amnions, one chorion and one placenta. Other types of multiple birth (triplets and so forth) may be derived from one or more zygotes.

Although the yolk sac and allantois are vestigial structures, their formation is essential for normal embryonic development. Both are important early sites of blood formation, and part of the yolk sac is incorporated into the embryo as the primitive gut. The amnion forms a sac for amniotic fluid and provides a covering for the umbilical cord. The amniotic fluid provides a protective buffer for the embryo, room for fetal movements and assistance in the regulation of fetal body temperature.

9

CONGENITAL MALFORMATIONS AND THEIR CAUSES

Not one of them is without meaning; not one that might not become the beginning of excellent knowledge, if only we could answer the question—why is it rare or being rare, why did it in this instance happen?

James Paget, 1882

Congenital malformations are anatomical or structural abnormalities present at birth. They may be macroscopic or microscopic, on the surface or within the body. About 15 per cent of deaths in the neonatal period* are attributed to congenital malformations. Congenital malformations are the largest single cause of severe illness and death during childhood. The branch of embryology dealing with abnormal development and congenital malformations is called *teratology*.

Although it is customary to divide the causes of congenital malformations into (1) *genetic factors* (chromosomal abnormalities or mutant genes) and (2) *environmental factors*, it is not usually possible to separate clearly the factors which cause the abnormalities. Most common malformations probably result from an interaction of genetic and environmental factors.

MALFORMATIONS CAUSED BY GENETIC FACTORS

Chromosomal abnormalities are present in about one of 200 newborn infants. Chromosome complements are subject to two kinds of changes: (1) numerical and (2) structural.

---

*The period just before and just after birth.

Numerical Chromosomal Abnormalities

Normally, the chromosomes exist in pairs; human females have 22 pairs of autosomes plus two X chromosomes, and males have 22 pairs of autosomes plus one X and one Y chromosome (Fig. 9–1). One of the two X chromosomes in female cells forms a mass of *sex chromatin* (Fig. 9–7B) which is not present in cells of normal males (Fig. 9–7A), or in those of females lacking a sex chromosome (Fig. 9–2).

Changes in chromosome number usually represent aneuploidy which is any deviation from the diploid number of 46 chromosomes. The cells may be hypodiploid (usually 45) or hyperdiploid (usually 47 to 49).

Monosomy. About 97 per cent of embryos lacking a sex chromosome die, but the remaining three per cent (about three in 10,000 newborn females) have characteristics of *Turner's syndrome* or *ovarian dysgenesis* (Fig. 9–2). Embryos missing an autosome or ordinary chromosome usually die; hence monosomy of an autosome is extremely rare in living persons.

Trisomy. If three chromosomes are present instead of the usual pair, the disorder is called trisomy. The usual cause of trisomy is nondisjunction or nonseparation

88

Autosomes

Sex Chromosomes

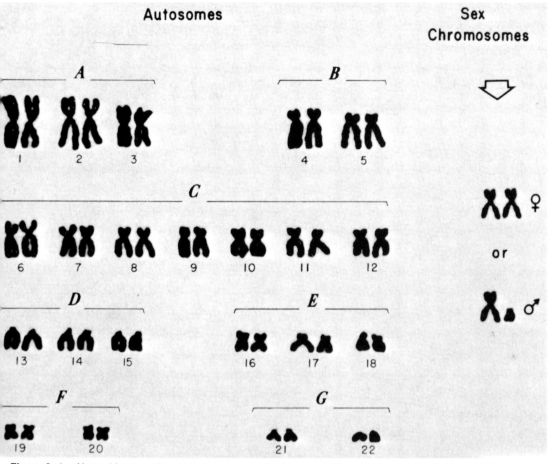

Figure 9–1. Normal human chromosomes arranged in the conventional manner known as a karyotype. The 44 autosomes are arranged in pairs in decreasing order of length and are divided into groups *A* to *G* on the basis of morphological similarities. The sex chromosomes are located on the right. (From Barr, M. L.: *Canad. Med. Ass. J. 95*:1137, 1966.)

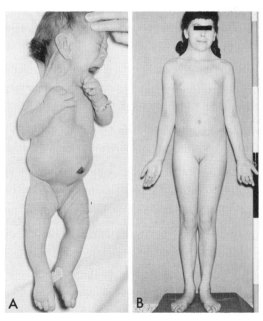

Figure 9–2. Females with Turner's syndrome and XO sex chromosome complement. *A,* Newborn infant. Note the webbed neck and lymphedema of the hands and feet. *B,* 13-year-old, showing the classic features. Note the short stature, webbed neck, absence of sexual maturation, and the broad shield-like chest with widely spaced nipples. (From Moore, K. L.: *The Sex Chromatin.* 1966. Courtesy of the W. B. Saunders Co.)

TABLE 9–1. TRISOMY OF THE AUTOSOMES

Disorder	Incidence	Usual Characteristics
21 trisomy or Down's syndrome*	1:600	Mental deficiency; flat nasal bridge; slant to palpebral fissures; protruding tongue; simian crease; congenital heart defects.
18 trisomy, E syndrome, or Edwards' syndrome†	1:3300	Mental deficiency; growth retardation; prominent occiput; short sternum; ventricular septal defect; micrognathia; low-set malformed ears; flexed fingers.
13–15 trisomy, D syndrome, or Patau's syndrome†	1:5500	Mental deficiency; sloping forehead; malformed ears; microphthalmos; bilateral cleft lip and/or palate; polydactyly; posterior prominence of the heels.

*The importance of this disorder in the overall problem of mental retardation is indicated by the fact that persons with Down's syndrome represent 10 to 15 per cent of institutionalized mental defectives.
†Infants with this syndrome rarely survive beyond a few months.

of chromosomes resulting in a germ cell with 24 instead of 23 chromosomes. If this cell is subsequently involved in fertilization, a zygote with 47 chromosomes forms.

Trisomy of the autosomes is primarily associated with three syndromes (Table 9–1). The most common condition is 21 trisomy or Down's syndrome (Fig. 9–3), in which three number 21 chromosomes are present; 18 trisomy (Fig. 9–4) and 13 to 15 trisomy (Fig. 9–5) are less common. Autosomal trisomies occur with increasing frequency as maternal age increases, particularly 21 trisomy, which is present once in about 2000 births in mothers under 25, but once in about 100 mothers over the age of 40.

Trisomy of the sex chromosomes is a relatively common condition (Table 9–2); however, because there are no characteristic physical findings in infants or children, it is rarely detected until adolescence or adulthood (Fig. 9–6). *Sex chromatin patterns* are useful in detecting trisomy of the sex chromosomes because two masses of sex chromatin are present in XXX females (Fig. 9–7C), and cells of XXY males are chromatin positive.

Tetrasomy and Pentasomy. Some persons, usually mentally retarded, have four or five sex chromosomes. Usually the greater the number of X chromosomes

present, the greater the severity of the mental retardation and physical impairment. The extra sex chromosomes do not accentuate male or female characteristics.

Structural Abnormalities

Most structural abnormalities result from environmental factors, e.g., radiation, drugs and viruses. The type of abnormality which results depends upon what happens to the broken pieces of chromosomes (Figs. 9–8 and 9–9).

Malformations Caused by Mutant Genes

About 10 to 15 per cent of congenital malformations are caused by mutant genes. Because these malformations are inherited according to Mendelian laws, predictions can be made about the probability of their occurrence in the affected person's children and other relatives. Although a great many genes mutate (undergo changes), most mutant genes do not cause congenital malformations. Examples of *dominantly inherited* congenital malformations are achondropla-

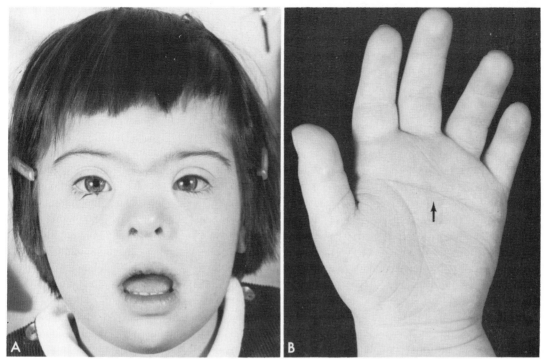

Figure 9–3. *A,* Photograph of a 3½-year-old girl, showing the typical facial appearance associated with Down's syndrome. Note the flat, broad face, oblique palpebral fissures, epicanthus, speckling of the iris and furrowed lower lip. *B,* The typical short, broad hand of this child shows the characteristic single transverse palmar or simian crease (arrow). (From Bartalos, M., and Baramki, T. A.: *Medical Cytogenetics.* 1967. Courtesy of the Williams & Wilkins Co.)

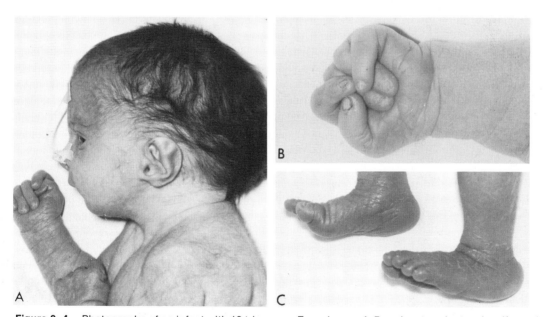

Figure 9–4. Photographs of an infant with 18 trisomy or E syndrome. *A,* Prominent occiput and malformed ears. *B,* Typical flexed fingers. *C,* So-called rocker-bottom feet, showing posterior prominences of the heels. (Courtesy of Dr. Harry Medovy, Children's Centre, Winnipeg.)

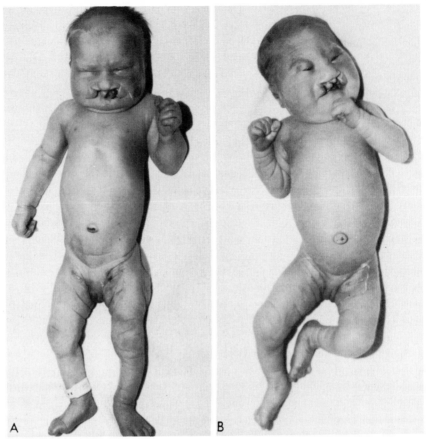

Figure 9–5. Female infants with 13–15 trisomy or D syndrome. Note bilateral cleft lip, sloping forehead and rocker-bottom feet. (From Smith, D. W.: *Amer. J. Obstet. Gynec. 90*:1055, 1964.)

TABLE 9–2. TRISOMY OF THE SEX CHROMOSOMES

Chromosome Complement*	Phenotype†	Incidence	Usual Characteristics
47,XXX	Female	1:1000	Normal in appearance; fertile; may be mentally retarded.
47,XXY	Male	1:500	Klinefelter's syndrome: small testes, hyalinization of seminiferous tubules, aspermatogenesis; may be mentally retarded.
47,XYY	Male	1:1000	Normal in appearance, often tall; may have personality disorder.

*The number designates the total number of chromosomes, including the sex chromosomes shown after the comma.

†A person's outward appearance resulting from his genetic constitution or genotype.

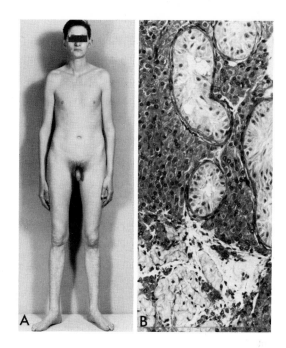

Figure 9-6. *A,* Adult male with XXY Klinefelter's syndrome. Note the relatively long legs and normal trunk length. *B,* Section of a testicular biopsy showing some seminiferous tubules without germ cells and others that are hyalinized. (From Ferguson-Smith, M. A.: *In* Moore, K. L. [Ed.]: *The Sex Chromatin.* 1966. Courtesy of the W. B. Saunders Co.)

sia (Fig. 9-10) and polydactyly or extra digits (see Chapter 16). Other malformations are attributed to *autosomal recessive inheritance,* e.g., microcephaly (see Chapter 17).

MALFORMATIONS CAUSED BY ENVIRONMENTAL FACTORS

The human embryo is well protected in the uterus, but certain agents or *teratogens* may induce congenital malformations. The embryonic organs are most sensitive to noxious agents during periods of rapid differentiation. Six mechanisms can cause congenital malformations: (1) too little growth, (2) too little resorption, (3) too much resorption, (4) resorption in the wrong location, (5) normal growth in an abnormal position, and (6) overgrowth of a tissue or structure.

Sensitive or Critical Periods. Environmental disturbances during the first two weeks after fertilization may interfere with implantation of the blastocyst or cause early death and abortion of the embryo. Development of the embryo is most easily disturbed during the *organogenetic period,* particularly from day 13 to 60. During this period, teratogenic agents are most likely to produce congenital malformations. Each organ has a critical period during which its development may be deranged (Fig. 9-11). Physiological defects, minor morphological abnormalities and functional disturbances, particularly of the central nervous system, are likely to result from disturbances during the fetal period.

Teratogens and Human Malformations

To prove that a given agent is teratogenic, one must show either that the frequency of malformations is increased above the "spontaneous" rate in pregnancies in which the mother is exposed to the agent (the prospective approach), or that malformed

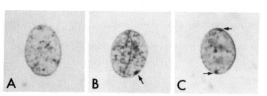

Figure 9-7. Oral epithelial nuclei stained with cresyl echt violet (×2000). *A,* From normal male. No sex chromatin is visible (chromatin negative). *B,* From normal female. The arrow indicates a typical mass of sex chromatin (chromatin positive). *C,* From female with XXX trisomy. The arrows indicate two masses of sex chromatin. (*A* and *B* are from Moore, K. L., and Barr, M. L.: *Lancet* 2:57, 1955.)

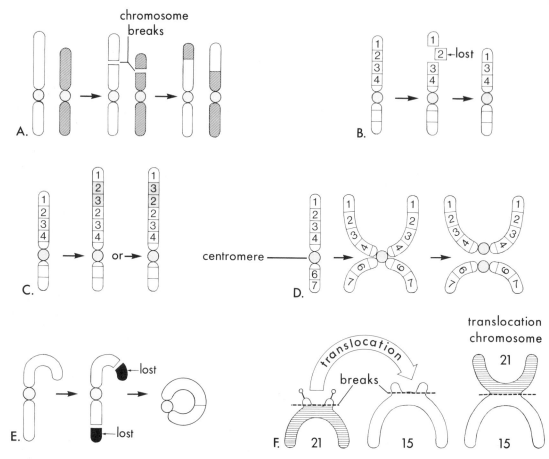

Figure 9–8. Diagrams illustrating structural abnormalities of chromosomes. *A*, Reciprocal translocation. *B*, Deletion. *C*, Duplication. *D*, Isochromosome. *E*, Ring chromosome. *F*, Translocation chromosome.

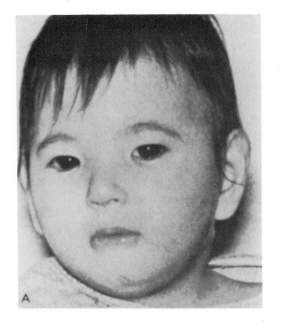

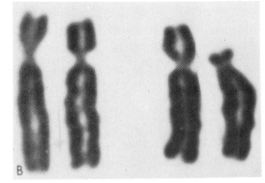

Figure 9–9. *A*, Male infant with cri du chat syndrome, showing the typical moon-faced appearance. *B*, The infant's B group of chromosomes (4 and 5), showing a deletion of chromosome number 5 on the right. (Courtesy of Dr. J. de Grouchy, Paris.)

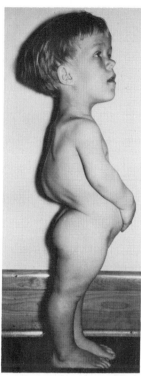

Figure 9–10. A child with achondroplasia, showing short extremities, relatively large head, thoracic kyphosis and protrusion of the abdomen. (Courtesy of Dr. Harry Medovy, Children's Centre, Winnipeg.)

children have a history of maternal exposure to the agent more often than normal children (the retrospective approach).

F. Clarke Fraser, 1967

Androgenic agents. The administration of synthetic progestins to prevent abortion has produced masculinization of female fetuses (Fig. 9–12 and Table 9–3).

Antibiotics. Tetracycline therapy during the second and third trimesters of pregnancy may cause minor tooth defects and discoloration of the deciduous or primary teeth. Penicillin appears to be harmless to the human embryo.

Antitumor agents. Tumor-inhibiting chemicals are highly teratogenic. *Aminopterin* is a potent teratogen which can induce major congenital malformations (Fig. 9–13), especially of the central nervous system. *Methotrexate*, a derivative of aminopterin, is also teratogenic.

Thyroid drugs. *Potassium iodide* and *radioactive iodine* may cause congenital goiter. Propylthiouracil interferes with thyroxin formation in the fetus and may cause goiter.

Thalidomide. A mass of evidence has shown that this drug is a potent teratogen. It has been estimated that 7000 infants were malformed by thalidomide (Fig. 9–14). The malformations ranged from amelia (absence of limbs) through intermediate stages of development (rudimentary limbs) to micromelia (short limbs). Thalidomide also causes malformations of other structures.

LSD and marijuana. There are conflicting views about the effects of LSD and marijuana on embryonic development. There is suggestive evidence that LSD may be teratogenic when taken during early human pregnancy; there have been reports of limb malformations and abnormalities of the central nervous system. Limb malformations have also been reported following the use of LSD and marijuana.

Drug testing in animals. Although the testing of drugs in pregnant animals is important, it should be emphasized that the results are of limited value for predicting drug effects on human embryos. Animal experiments can only suggest similar effects in man.

Infectious Agents

There is convincing proof that three microorganisms (rubella virus, cytomegalovirus and *Toxoplasma gondii*) cause congenital malformations.

Rubella (German Measles). About 15 to 20 per cent of infants born to women who have had German measles during the first trimester of pregnancy are congenitally malformed. The usual triad of malformations is *cataract* (Fig. 9–15*A*), *cardiac malformations* and *deafness*. The earlier in pregnancy the maternal rubella infection occurs, the greater is the danger of the embryo being malformed. Most infants have congenital malformations if the disease occurs during the first five weeks after fertilization. This is understandable because this period includes the most susceptible organogenetic periods of the eye, ear, heart and brain (Fig. 9–11). Malformations may result from infections during the second and third trimesters, but usually functional defects of the central nervous system and ear result.

Cytomegalovirus. Infection with this virus during the second and third trimesters causes abnormalities of the brain (microcephaly) and of the eyes (microphthalmia).

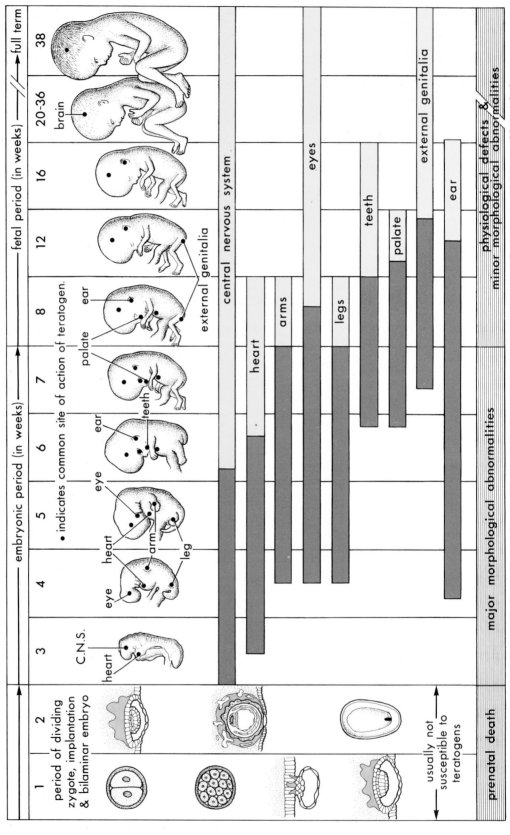

Figure 9–11. Schematic illustration of the sensitive or critical periods in human development. Red denotes highly sensitive periods; yellow indicates stages that are less sensitive to teratogens.

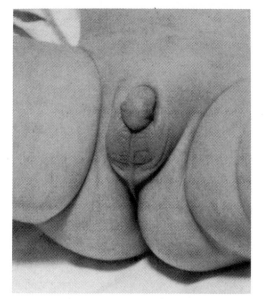 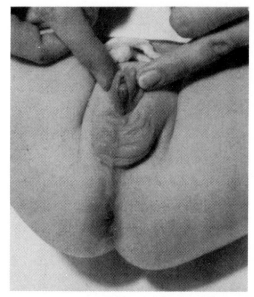

Figure 9–12. The external genitalia of a newborn female infant showing labial fusion and enlargement of the clitoris caused by an androgenic agent given to the infant's mother during the first trimester. (From Jones, H. W., and Scott, W. W.: *Hermaphroditism, Genital Anomalies and Related Endocrine Disorders.* 1958. Courtesy of the Williams & Wilkins Co.)

Toxoplasma gondii. This intracellular parasite can be contracted from eating raw or poorly cooked meat, or by contact with infected animals. This organism may cross the placental membrane and infect the fetus, causing destructive changes in the brain and eye, resulting in microcephaly, microphthalmia and hydrocephaly (see Chapters 17 and 18).

Irradiation

Ionizing radiations are potent teratogens. Treatment of pregnant mothers during the

TABLE 9–3. TERATOGENS KNOWN TO CAUSE HUMAN MALFORMATIONS

Teratogens	Malformations

Androgenic Agents
  Ethisterone
  Norethisterone
	Varying degrees of masculinization of female fetuses: most have labial fusion and clitoral hypertrophy.

Antitumor Agents Aminopterin	Wide range of skeletal defects and malformations of the central nervous system, notably anencephaly.
Bulsulfan (Myleran) alternating with 6-mercaptopurine	Stunted growth, skeletal abnormalities, corneal opacities, cleft palate and hypoplasia of various organs.
Methotrexate	Multiple malformations, especially skeletal.
Thalidomide	Meromelia and other limb malformations, external ear, cardiac and gastrointestinal malformations.
Infectious Agents Cytomegalovirus	Microcephaly, hydrocephaly, and mental retardation (see Chapter 17).
Rubella virus	Cataract, deafness, and congenital heart defects.
Toxoplasma gondii	Microcephaly, microphthalmia, hydrocephaly and chorioretinitis.
Therapeutic Radiation	Microcephaly and skeletal malformations.

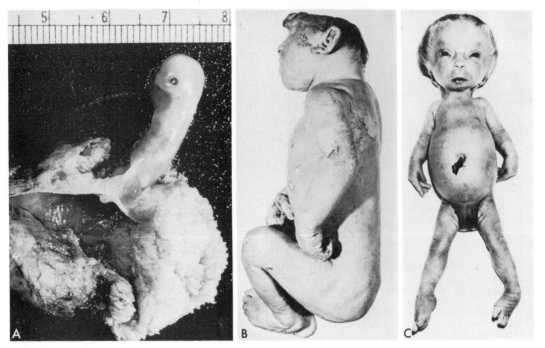

Figure 9-13. Aminopterin-induced congenital malformations. *A,* Grossly malformed embryo and its membranes. (Courtesy of Dr. J. B. Thiersch, Seattle, Washington.) *B,* Newborn infant with anencephaly or partial absence of the brain. (From Thiersch, J. B., *in* Wolstenholme, G. E. W., and O'Connor, C. M. [Eds.]: *Ciba Foundation Symposium on Congenital Malformations.* London, J. & A. Churchill, Ltd., 1960, pp. 152–154.) *C,* Newborn infant showing marked intrauterine growth retardation (2380 gm), a large head, a small mandible, deformed ears, clubhands and clubfeet. (From Warkany, J., Beaudry, P. H., and Hornstein, S.: *Amer. J. Dis. Child. 97:*274, 1960.)

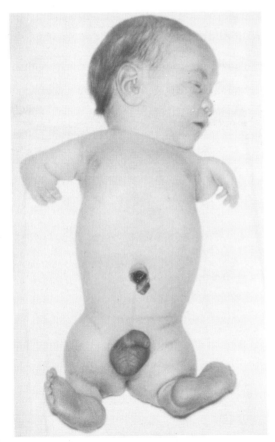

Figure 9-14. Newborn male infant showing typically malformed limbs (meromelia) caused by thalidomide. (From Moore, K. L.: *Manitoba Med. Rev. 43:*306, 1963.)

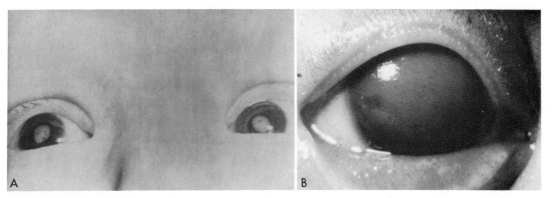

Figure 9–15. Congenital malformations of the eye caused by the rubella virus. *A,* Cataracts. (From Cooper, L. Z., *et al.: Amer. J. Dis. Child. 110*:416, 1965. Courtesy of Dr. Richard Baragry, Department of Ophthalmology, Cornell-New York Hospital.) *B,* Glaucoma. (From Cooper, L. Z., *et al.: Amer. J. Dis. Child. 110*:416, 1965. Courtesy of Dr. Daniel I. Weiss, Department of Ophthalmology, New York University School of Medicine.)

embryo's susceptible period of development with large doses of roentgen rays and radium may cause microcephaly, mental retardation and skeletal malformations.

There is no proof that congenital malformations have been caused by diagnostic X-rays, but there are grounds for caution especially during the first trimester.

SUMMARY

Much progress has been made in recent years in the search for causes of congenital malformations, but satisfactory explanations are still lacking for most of them. Developmental abnormalities may be macroscopic or microscopic, on the surface or within the body. Some congenital malformations are caused by *genetic factors* (chromosomal abnormalities and mutant genes) and a few are caused by *environmental factors* (infectious agents and teratogenic drugs), but most common malformations result from a complex interaction of genetic and environmental factors.

During the first two weeks of development, teratogenic agents may kill the embryo or cause chromosomal abnormalities which give rise to congenital malformations. During the *organogenetic period*, particularly from day 13 to 60, teratogenic agents may cause major congenital malformations. During the fetal period, teratogens may produce minor morphological and functional abnormalities, particularly of the brain and the eyes. However, it must be stressed that some drugs and infections may adversely affect the fetus without causing congenital malformations.

10

BODY CAVITIES AND THE DIAPHRAGM

Early development of the intraembryonic coelom or embryonic body cavity is described in Chapter 5. By the fourth week it appears as a horseshoe-shaped cavity (Fig. 10–1A). The curve of the "horseshoe" represents the future *pericardial cavity*, and the lateral extensions indicate the future *pleural* and *peritoneal cavities*. The intraembryonic coelom provides room for organ development and movement. For a while the intraembryonic coelom communicates with the extraembryonic coelom at the lateral edges of the embryonic disc (Fig. 10–1A and B). This communication is largely occluded during folding of the embryonic disc into a cylindrical embryo, but persists for awhile around the stalk of the yolk sac (Fig. 10–2E).

During transverse folding of the embryo, the lateral extensions of the intraembryonic coelom come together and fuse on the ventral aspect of the embryo (Fig. 10–2C and F). In the region of the future peritoneal cavity, the ventral mesentery degenerates, forming a large embryonic cavity extending from the thoracic to the pelvic region. Three body cavities now recognizable are : (1) a large *pericardial cavity* around the heart (Fig. 10–2B and E); (2) two relatively small pericardioperitoneal canals (or pleural

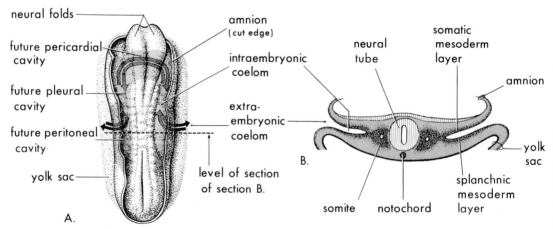

Figure 10–1. *A*, Embryo of about 22 days showing the outline of the horseshoe-shaped intraembryonic coelom. The amnion has been removed and the coelom is shown as if the embryo were translucent. The continuity of the coelom and the communication of its right and left extremities with the extraembryonic coelom is indicated by arrows. *B*, Transverse section through the embryo at the level shown in *A*.

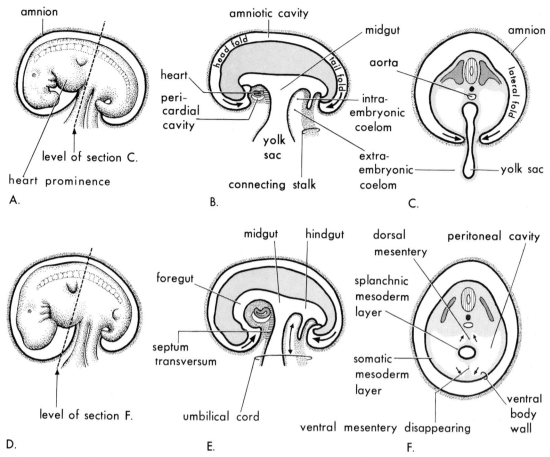

Figure 10–2. Drawings illustrating folding of the embryo and its effects on the intraembryonic coelom and other structures. *A*, Lateral view of an embryo of about 26 days. *B*, Schematic longitudinal section of this embryo showing the head and tail folds. *C*, Transverse section at the level shown in *A* indicating how the lateral folds give the embryo a cylindrical form. *D*, Lateral view of a 28-day embryo. *E*, Schematic longitudinal section of this embryo showing the reduced communication between the intraembryonic and extraembryonic coeloms or cavities (double-headed arrow). *F*, Transverse section as indicated in *D*, illustrating formation of the ventral body wall and disappearance of the ventral mesentery. The arrows indicate the junction of the somatic and splanchnic mesoderm layers.

canals) connecting the pericardial and peritoneal cavities (Fig. 10–3) containing the abdominal and pelvic viscera (Fig. 10–2*F*).

With formation of the head fold, the heart and pericardial cavity move or "swing" ventrally beneath the foregut (Fig. 10–2*B* and *E*). The pericardial cavity then opens dorsally into the pericardioperitoneal canals, which pass dorsal to the septum transversum on each side of the foregut (Fig. 10–3). The *septum transversum* is a transverse sheet of mesoderm which separates the pericardial cavity from the peritoneal cavity, forming a partial diaphragm or partition between them.

DIVISION OF THE COELOM

Partitions form at both ends of the pericardioperitoneal canals and separate the pericardial cavity from the pleural cavities, and the pleural cavities from the peritoneal cavity.

The *pleuropericardial membranes* separate the pericardial cavity from the pleural cavities. Initially, this pair of membranes appears as ridges or bulges containing the *common cardinal veins* on their way to the heart (Fig. 10–4*A*). At first the pleuropericardial membranes are free dorsally and project into the cranial ends of the pericardioperi-

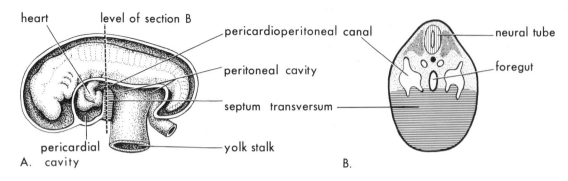

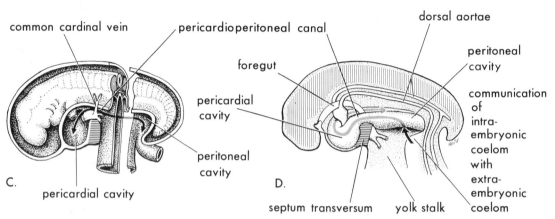

Figure 10–3. Schematic drawings of a four-week embryo. *A,* The lateral wall of the pericardial cavity has been removed to show the heart. *B,* Transverse section illustrating the relationship of the pericardioperitoneal canals to the septum transversum (partial diaphragm) and the foregut. *C,* Lateral view with the heart removed. The embryo has been sectioned transversely to show the continuity of the intraembryonic and extraembryonic coeloms or body cavities. *D,* Sketch showing the pericardioperitoneal canals arising from the dorsal wall of the pericardial cavity and passing on each side of the foregut to join the peritoneal cavity. The arrows show the communication of the extraembryonic coelom with the intraembryonic coelom and the continuity of the intra-embryonic coelom.

toneal canals; however, after expansion of the pleural cavities, the pleuropericardial membranes fuse with one another and with the mesoderm ventral to the esophagus (Fig. 10–4C).

The *pleuroperitoneal membranes* separate the pleural cavities from the peritoneal cavity (Fig. 10–5). These membranes project into the caudal ends of the pericardioperitoneal canals (Fig. 10–5B), and later fuse with other diaphragmatic components to form the diaphragm (Fig. 10–5C to E).

DEVELOPMENT OF THE DIAPHRAGM

This diaphragm is a dome-shaped musculotendinous partition separating the thoracic and abdominopelvic cavities. It mainly develops from four structures (Fig. 10–5).

The Septum Transversum. This structure initially forms a thick incomplete partition or partial diaphragm between the pericardial and peritoneal cavities (Fig. 10–3). Later it fuses dorsally with the mesoderm ventral to the esophagus and with the pleuroperitoneal membranes (Fig. 10–5C). Eventually, it forms the *central tendon* of the adult diaphragm (Fig. 10–5E).

The Pleuroperitoneal Membranes. These membranes fuse with the dorsal mesentery of the esophagus and with the dorsal portion of the septum transversum (Fig. 10–5C), thereby completing the partition between the thoracic and abdominopelvic cavities. Although the pleuroperitoneal membranes form large portions of the primitive

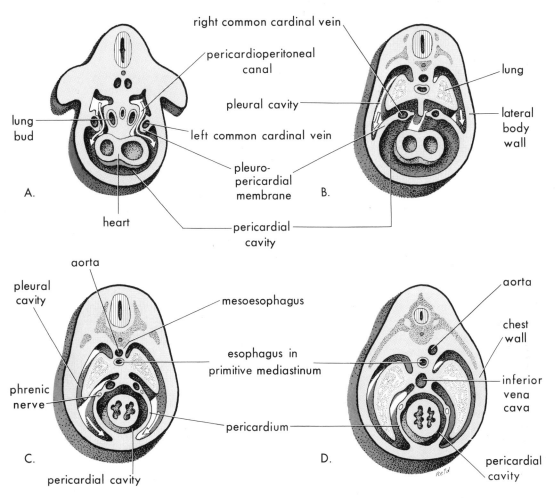

Figure 10–4. Schematic drawings of transverse sections through an embryo cranial to the septum transversum, illustrating successive stages in the separation of the pleural cavities from the pericardial cavity. Growth and development of the lungs, expansion of the pleural cavities and formation of the fibrous pericardium are also shown. *A*, Five weeks. The arrows indicate the communications between the pericardioperitoneal canals and the pericardial cavity. *B*, Six weeks. The arrows indicate development of the pleural cavities as extensions of the pericardioperitoneal canals and expansion of the pleural cavities into the body wall. *C*, Seven weeks. Expansion of the pleural cavities ventrally around the heart is shown. The pleuropericardial membranes are now fused in the midline with each other and with the mesoderm ventral to the esophagus. *D*, Eight weeks. Continued expansion of the lungs and pleural cavities and formation of the fibrous pericardium and chest wall are illustrated.

diaphragm, they represent relatively small intermediate portions of the final diaphragm (Fig. 10–5*E*).

Dorsal Mesentery of the Esophagus. This mesentery constitutes the median portion of the diaphragm (Fig. 10–5*E*).

The Body Wall. As the lungs grow, the pleural cavities enlarge and burrow into the lateral body walls (Figs. 10–4 and 10–5*B* to

D). During this "excavation" process, body-wall tissue is split off and forms peripheral portions of the diaphragm.

Congenital Diaphragmatic Hernia

A posterolateral defect of the diaphragm is a relatively common developmental ab-

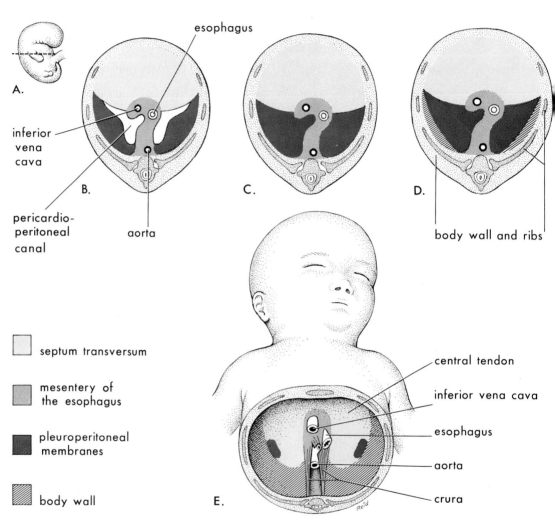

esophagus

A.

inferior
vena
cava

B.

C.

D.

pericardio-
peritoneal
canal

aorta

body wall and ribs

septum transversum

mesentery of
the esophagus

pleuroperitoneal
membranes

body wall

E.

central tendon

inferior vena cava

esophagus

aorta

crura

Figure 10–5. Drawings illustrating development of the diaphragm as viewed from below. *A,* Sketch of a lateral view of an embryo at the end of the fifth week (*actual size*) indicating the level of section *B. B,* Transverse section showing the unfused pleuroperitoneal membranes. *C,* Similar section at the end of the sixth week after fusion of the pleuroperitoneal membranes with the other two diaphragmatic components. *D,* Transverse section through a 12-week embryo after ingrowth of the fourth diaphragmatic component from the body wall. *E,* View of the diaphragm of a newborn infant, indicating the probable embryological origin of its components.

vertebra   defect

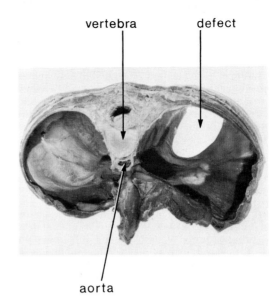

Figure 10-6. Photograph of a transverse section through the thoracic region of a newborn infant, viewed from above. Note the large left posterolateral defect of the diaphragm. *Half actual size.*

aorta

normality (Fig. 10–6). It results from failure of the pleuroperitoneal membrane on the affected side to fuse with other diaphragmatic components. The defect consists of a large opening in the posterolateral region of the diaphragm, usually in the region of the left kidney. There is free communication between the abdominal and pleural cavities. As a result, the intestines and other abdominal organs pass into the thorax.

SUMMARY

The intraembryonic coelom or embryonic body cavity begins to develop near the end of the third week. Later it appears as a continuous horseshoe-shaped cavity. During folding of the embryonic disc in the fourth week, the lateral extensions of the coelom are brought together on the ventral aspect of the embryo, where they fuse in the region of the future peritoneal cavity.

Until the seventh week, the pericardial cavity communicates with the peritoneal cavity through paired pericardioperitoneal canals. During the fifth and sixth weeks, partitions or membranes form at the cranial and caudal ends of these canals. The cranial pleuropericardial membranes separate the pericardial cavity from the pleural cavities, and the caudal pleuroperitoneal membranes separate the pleural cavities from the peritoneal cavity.

The diaphragm develops from four main structures: (1) the septum transversum, (2) the pleuroperitoneal membranes, (3) the dorsal mesentery of the esophagus, and (4) the body wall. Posterolateral defect of the diaphragm is the commonest type of congenital diaphragmatic defect and is associated with herniation of abdominal viscera into the thoracic cavity.

11

THE BRANCHIAL APPARATUS AND ITS DERIVATIVES

The branchial apparatus consists of (1) *pharyngeal* or *branchial arches*, (2) *pharyngeal pouches*, (3) *branchial grooves* or *clefts*, and (4) *branchial* or *closing membranes* (Fig. 11–1). The cranial region of an early human embryo somewhat resembles a fish embryo of a comparable stage, but these ancestral structures become rearranged and adapted to new functions or disappear.

THE BRANCHIAL ARCHES

Branchial arches develop during the fourth week and appear as ridges on the future head and neck region (Fig. 11–1B to G). The arches are separated from each other by *branchial grooves* or clefts (Fig. 11–1D). They are numbered in a craniocaudal sequence.

The mouth initially appears as a slight depression of the surface ectoderm, called the *stomodeum* or *primitive mouth* (Fig. 11–1D to G). At first this cavity is separated from the foregut or primitive pharynx by a bilaminar membrane, the *oropharyngeal* or *buccopharyngeal membrane*. This membrane ruptures at about 24 days, bringing the digestive tract into communication with the amniotic cavity.

Fate of the Branchial Arches. The first branchial arch is involved with development of the face and is subsequently discussed with this region. During the fifth week, the

second (hyoid) arch overgrows the third and fourth arches, forming an ectodermal depression known as the *cervical sinus* (Fig. 11–3A to D). During the sixth and seventh weeks, the second and sixth arches enlarge and merge with each other. Gradually, the second to fourth branchial grooves and the cervical sinus are obliterated, giving the neck a smooth contour (Fig. 11–3F and G). The branchial arches caudal to the second one make little contribution to the skin of the neck (Fig. 11–3G).

Derivatives of the Branchial Arch Cartilages (Fig. 11–4). The dorsal end of the *first arch cartilage*, or *Meckel's cartilage*, becomes ossified to form two middle ear bones, the *malleus* and the *incus*. The intermediate portion of the cartilage regresses, and its perichondrium forms the *anterior ligament of the malleus* and the *sphenomandibular ligament*. The ventral portion of Meckel's cartilage largely disappears; the mandible develops around it by intramembranous ossification.

The dorsal end of the *second arch cartilage*, or *Reichert's cartilage*, also ossifies and forms the stapes of the middle ear and the *styloid process* of the temporal bone. The portion of cartilage between the styloid process and the hyoid bone regresses, and its perichondrium forms the *stylohyoid ligament*. The ventral end of Reichert's cartilage ossifies to form the lesser cornu and upper part of the body of the *hyoid bone*.

The *third arch cartilage* is located in the

(Text continued on page 110.)

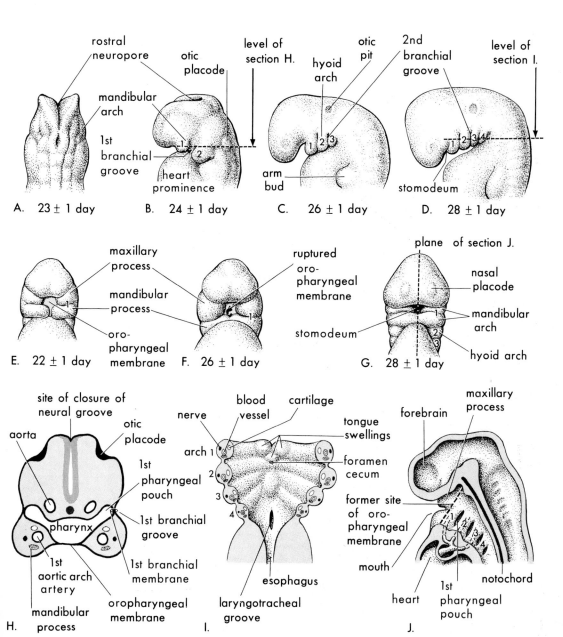

Figure 11–1. Drawings illustrating the human branchial apparatus. *A*, Dorsal view of the cranial part of an early embryo. *B* to *D*, Lateral views, showing later development of the branchial arches. *E* to *G*, Facial views, illustrating the relationship of the first arch to the stomodeum or primitive mouth. *H*, Transverse section through the cranial region of an embryo. *I*, Horizontal section through the cranial region of an embryo, illustrating the branchial arch components and the floor of the primitive pharynx. *J*, Sagittal section of the upper region of an embryo, illustrating the openings of the pharyngeal pouches in the lateral wall of the primitive pharynx.

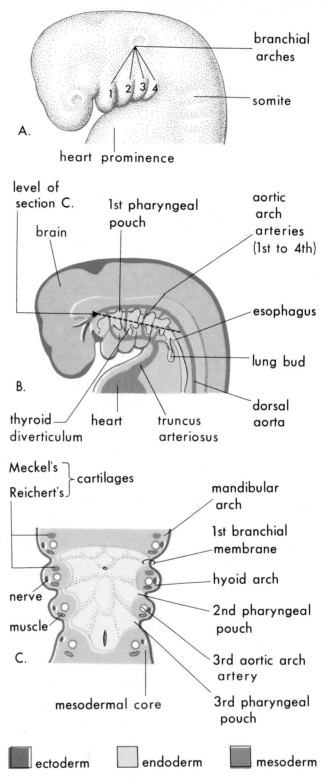

Figure 11–2. *A,* Drawing of the head and neck region of a 28-day embryo. *B,* Schematic drawing showing the pharyngeal pouches and aortic or branchial arch arteries, exposed by removal of the ectoderm and mesoderm. *C,* Horizontal section through the embryo, illustrating the germ layer of origin of the branchial arch components.

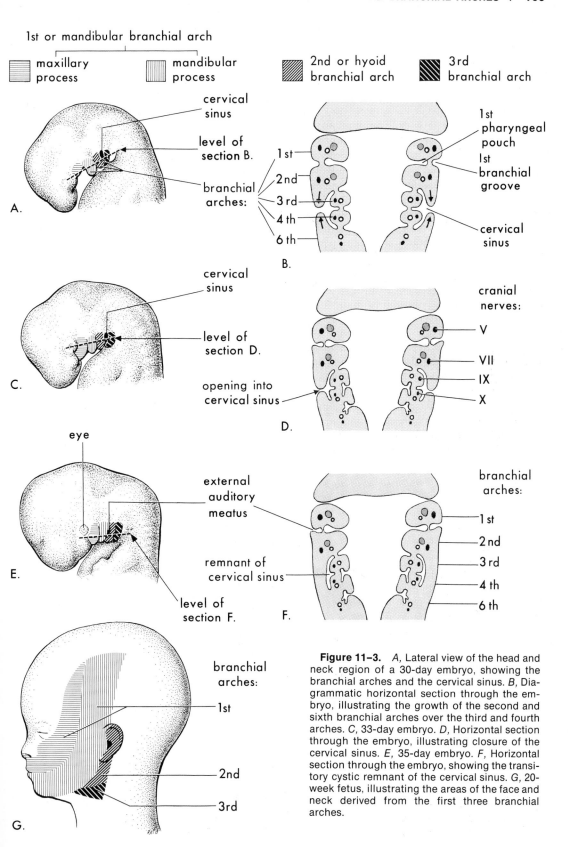

1st or mandibular branchial arch

maxillary process

mandibular process

2nd or hyoid branchial arch

3rd branchial arch

A.

cervical sinus

level of section B.

branchial arches:

1st
2nd
3rd
4th
6th

B.

1st pharyngeal pouch

1st branchial groove

cervical sinus

C.

cervical sinus

level of section D.

opening into cervical sinus

D.

cranial nerves:

V
VII
IX
X

E.

eye

external auditory meatus

remnant of cervical sinus

level of section F.

F.

branchial arches:

1st
2nd
3rd
4th
6th

G.

branchial arches:

1st
2nd
3rd

Figure 11–3. *A,* Lateral view of the head and neck region of a 30-day embryo, showing the branchial arches and the cervical sinus. *B,* Diagrammatic horizontal section through the embryo, illustrating the growth of the second and sixth branchial arches over the third and fourth arches. *C,* 33-day embryo. *D,* Horizontal section through the embryo, illustrating closure of the cervical sinus. *E,* 35-day embryo. *F,* Horizontal section through the embryo, showing the transitory cystic remnant of the cervical sinus. *G,* 20-week fetus, illustrating the areas of the face and neck derived from the first three branchial arches.

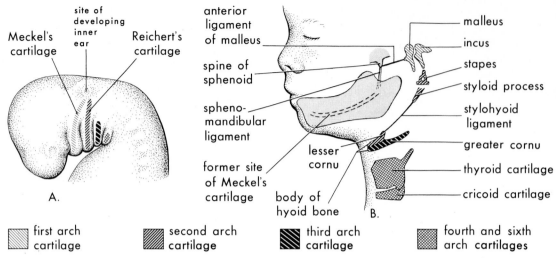

first arch cartilage

second arch cartilage

third arch cartilage

fourth and sixth arch cartilages

Figure 11-4. *A,* Schematic lateral view of the head and neck region of a four-week embryo, illustrating the location of the branchial arch cartilages. *B,* Similar view of a 24-week fetus, illustrating the adult derivatives of the branchial arch cartilages.

ventral portion of the arch and ossifies to from the greater cornu and lower part of the body of the hyoid bone. The *fourth, fifth and sixth arch cartilages* are in the ventral regions of the arches; they form the *laryngeal cartilages.*

Derivatives of the Branchial Arch Muscles (Fig. 11-5). The muscle elements in the

branchial arches form various striated muscles in the head and neck.

THE PHARYNGEAL POUCHES

The primitive pharynx is wide cranially and narrow caudally. The endoderm of the

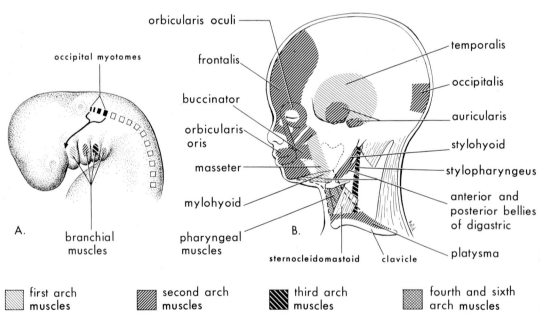

first arch muscles

second arch muscles

third arch muscles

fourth and sixth arch muscles

Figure 11-5. *A,* Sketch of lateral view of the head and neck region of a four-week embryo, showing the branchial muscles. The arrow shows the pathway taken by myoblasts from the occipital myotomes to form the tongue musculature. *B,* Sketch of the head and neck of a 20-week fetus dissected to show the muscles derived from the branchial arches. Parts of the platysma and sternocleidomastoid muscles have been removed to show the deeper muscles.

pharynx lines the inner aspects of the branchial arches and passes into balloon-like outgrowths called *pharyngeal pouches* (Figs. 11–1*H* to *J* and 11–2*B* and *C*). The pouches develop in a craniocaudal sequence between the branchial arches, e.g., the first pouch lies between the first and second branchial arches. There are four well-defined pairs of pouches.

Derivatives of the Pharyngeal Pouches

The First Pharyngeal Pouch. This pouch expands into an elongate *tubotympanic recess* which forms the *tympanic cavity and antrum*. Its connection with the pharynx gradually elongates to form the pharyngotympanic (Eustachian) tube (Fig. 11–6).

The Second Pharyngeal Pouch. The endoderm of this pouch proliferates and forms buds. The central parts of these buds break down, forming the tonsillar *crypts*. The pouch endoderm forms the surface epithelium and the lining of the *crypts of the palatine tonsil*. The mesenchyme surrounding the crypts differentiates into lymphoid tissue and soon becomes organized into *lymph nodules*.

The Third Pharyngeal Pouch. This pouch expands into a solid dorsal bulbar portion and a hollow ventral elongate part. Each dorsal bulbar portion differentiates into an *inferior parathyroid gland*. The elongate ventral portions form two pouches that eventually meet and fuse to form the thymus. The *thymus* and parathyroid glands migrate caudally. Later the parathyroid glands separate from the thymus and come to lie on the dorsal surface of the thyroid gland which has descended from the foramen cecum of the tongue (Fig. 11–6*C*).

The Fourth Pharyngeal Pouch. This pouch also expands into a dorsal bulbar portion and a ventral elongate part. Each dorsal portion develops into a *superior parathyroid gland*. The ventral elongate part of each fourth pouch develops into an *ultimobranchial body* which becomes incorporated into the thyroid gland and gives rise to the *parafollicular* or *C cells*. These cells produce *thyrocalcitonin*, a hormone involved in the regulation of the normal calcium level in body fluids.

The Fifth Pharyngeal Pouch. This is a rudimentary structure which is partially incorporated into the fourth pouch.

The Thyroid Gland

The thyroid gland appears during the third week as a median endodermal thickening in the floor of the primitive pharynx (Fig. 11–7). This thickening soon becomes a downgrowth known as the *thyroid diverticulum* (Figs. 11–2*B*, 11–6*A* and 11–7*A*). The developing thyroid descends in the front of the neck, retaining its connection to the tongue by a narrow *thyroglossal duct* (Fig. 11–7*B* and *C*). This duct's opening in the tongue is called the *foramen cecum*. By seven weeks the thyroid gland has usually reached its final site in front of the trachea, and the thyroglossal duct has normally disappeared. The original opening of the thyroglossal duct persists as a vestigial pit, the foramen cecum of the tongue (Figs. 11–7*D* and 11–8*C*).

The Tongue

The first indication of tongue development appears around the end of the fourth week as a median elevation, the *tuberculum impar* (median tongue bud or swelling), in the floor of the pharynx just cranial to the foramen cecum (Fig. 11–8*A*). Two oval *lateral lingual swellings* (distal tongue buds or swellings) soon develop on each side of the tuberculum impar. The lateral lingual swellings rapidly increase in size, merge with each other and overgrow the tuberculum impar. The fused lateral lingual swellings form the *anterior two-thirds*, or *body*, of the tongue (Fig. 11–8*C*).

The *posterior third*, or *root*, of the tongue is initially indicated by two elevations that develop caudal to the foramen cecum (Fig. 11–8*A*). One, the *copula* (connector), is formed by fusion of the ventromedial parts of the second branchial arches; the other, called the *hypobranchial eminence*, develops caudal to the copula from mesoderm in the ventromedial parts of the third and fourth branchial arches.

(Text continued on page 115.)

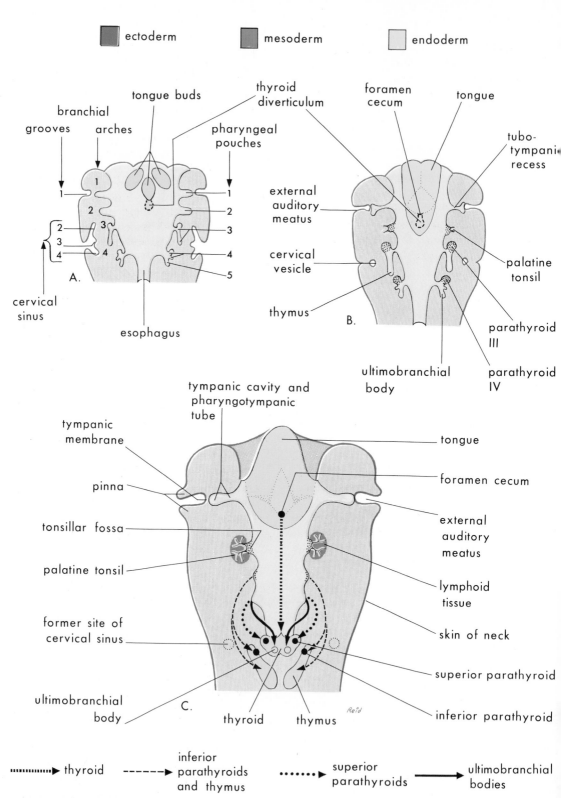

Figure 11-6. Schematic horizontal sections at the level shown in Figure 11-3A, illustrating the adult derivatives of the pharyngeal pouches. A, Five weeks. B, Six weeks. C, Seven weeks.

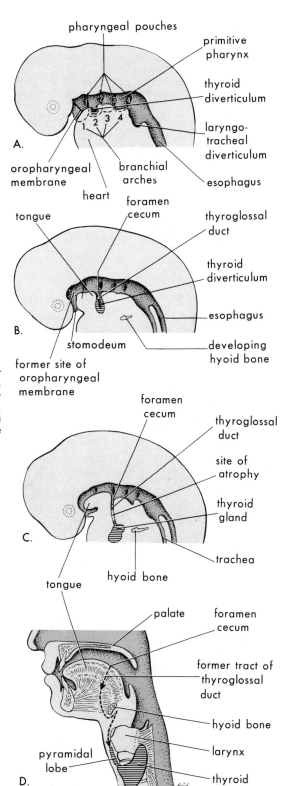

Figure 11–7. *A, B* and *C*, Schematic sagittal sections of the head and neck region of embryos at four, five and six weeks, respectively, illustrating successive stages of development of the thyroid gland. *D,* Similar section of an adult head, showing the path taken by the thyroid gland during its descent and the former tract of the thyroglossal duct.

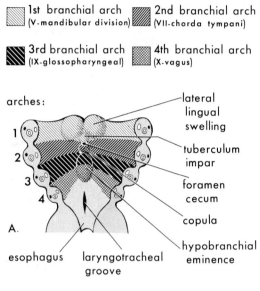

1st branchial arch
(V-mandibular division)

2nd branchial arch
(VII-chorda tympani)

3rd branchial arch
(IX-glossopharyngeal)

4th branchial arch
(X-vagus)

arches:

1
2
3
4

A.

lateral lingual swelling

tuberculum impar

foramen cecum

copula

hypobranchial eminence

esophagus   laryngotracheal groove

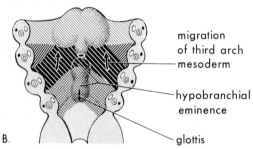

B.

migration of third arch mesoderm

hypobranchial eminence

glottis

Figure 11-8. *A* and *B,* Schematic horizontal sections through the pharynx at the level shown in Figure 11-3*A,* showing successive stages in the development of the tongue during the fourth and fifth weeks. *C,* Adult tongue showing the branchial arch derivation of the nerve supply of the mucosa.

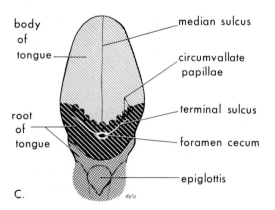

body of tongue

root of tongue

C.

median sulcus

circumvallate papillae

terminal sulcus

foramen cecum

epiglottis

As the tongue develops, the copula is gradually overgrown by the hypobranchial eminence (Fig. 11–8*B* and *C*). As a result, the posterior third of the tongue develops from the cranial part of the hypobranchial eminence. The line of fusion of the anterior and posterior parts of the tongue is roughly indicated by the V-shaped groove called the *terminal sulcus* (Fig. 11–8*C*).

DEVELOPMENT OF THE FACE

The *five facial primordia* appear around the stomodeum or primitive mouth early in the fourth week (Fig. 11–9*A*): The large *frontonasal elevation* or process constitutes the upper boundary of the stomodeum. The paired *maxillary processes* of the first branchial arch form the lateral boundaries or sides of the stomodeum. The paired *mandibular processes* of this same arch constitute the lower boundary of the stomodeum.

Bilateral oval-shaped thickenings of the surface ectoderm, called *nasal placodes*, develop on each side of the lower part of frontonasal elevation (Fig. 11–9*B*). Horseshoe-shaped *medial and lateral nasal elevations* or processes develop at the margins of the nasal placodes (Fig. 11–9*C* and *D*). As a result, the nasal placodes lie in depressions called *nasal pits* (Fig. 11–9*C*). The maxillary processes grow rapidly and soon approach each other and the medial nasal elevations (Fig. 11–9*D* and *E*).

During the sixth and seventh weeks, the medial nasal elevations merge with each other and the maxillary processes (Fig. 11–9*F* and *G*). As the medial nasal elevations merge with each other, they form an *intermaxillary segment* of the upper jaw (Fig. 11–9*H*). This segment gives rise to (1) the middle portion of the upper lip called the *philtrum*; (2) the middle portion of the upper jaw and its associated gingiva (gum); and (3) the *primary palate*.

The lateral parts of the upper lip, the upper jaw and the secondary palate form from the maxillary processes (Figs. 11–9*H* and *I* and 11–10). These processes merge laterally with the mandibular processes and reduce the size of the mouth. The *frontonasal elevation* forms the forehead and the dorsum and apex of the nose. The sides or ala of the nose are derived from the lateral nasal elevations (Fig. 11–9*H* and *I*).

The mandibular processes merge with each other in the fourth week and the groove between them disappears before the end of the fifth week (Fig. 11–9*D*). The mandibular processes give rise to the lower jaw, the lower lip and the lower part of the face. Final development of the face occurs slowly and results mainly from changes in the proportion and relative position of the facial components.

DEVELOPMENT OF THE PALATE

The palate develops from the *primary palate* and the *secondary palate*.

The Primary Palate. The primary palate, or median palatine process, develops at the end of the fifth week from the innermost part of the intermaxillary segment of the upper jaw. It forms a wedge-shaped mass of mesoderm between the maxillary processes of the developing upper jaw (Fig. 11–10*F*).

The Secondary Palate. The secondary palate develops from two horizontal projections from the maxillary processes, called the *lateral palatine processes* (Fig. 11–10*B*). They initially project downward on each side of the tongue (Fig. 11–10*C*), but as the jaws develop, the tongue moves downward and the lateral palatine processes gradually grow toward each other and fuse (Fig. 11–10*E* and *G*). They also fuse with the primary palate and the *nasal septum* (Fig. 11–10*D* to *H*). The fusion begins anteriorly during the ninth week and is complete posteriorly by the twelfth week. The uvula (Latin, meaning "little grape") is the last part of the palate to form. The *palatine raphe* indicates the line of fusion of the lateral palatine processes (Fig. 11–10*H*).

CONGENITAL MALFORMATIONS OF THE HEAD AND NECK

Abnormalities of the head and neck mainly originate during transformation of the branchial apparatus into adult structures. Malformations associated with transformation of the aortic arch system of the branchial arches into the adult arterial pattern are described in Chapter 15.

Congenital Auricular Pits and Cysts. Small blind pits or cysts in the skin are commonly found in a triangular area anterior to the ear (Fig. 11–11*F*). Although often claimed

(Text continued on page 120.)

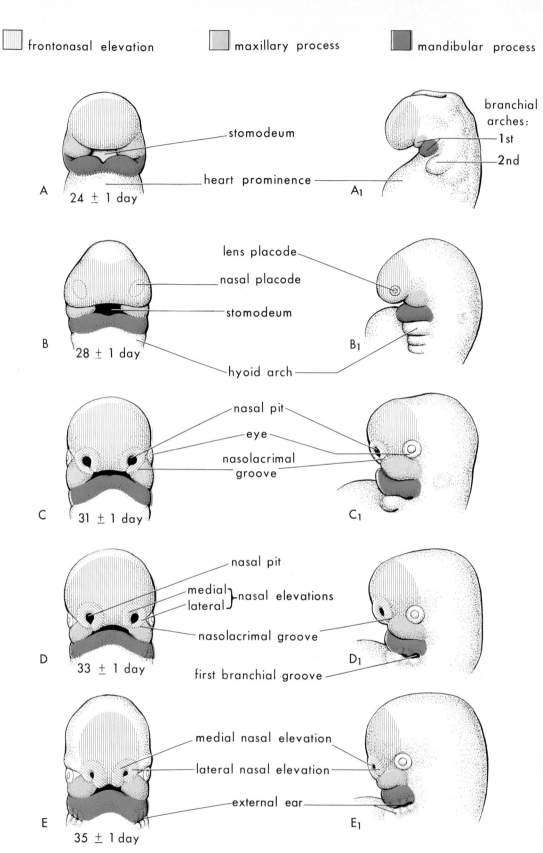

Figure 11–9. Diagrams illustrating progressive stages in the development of the human face during the embryonic and fetal periods.

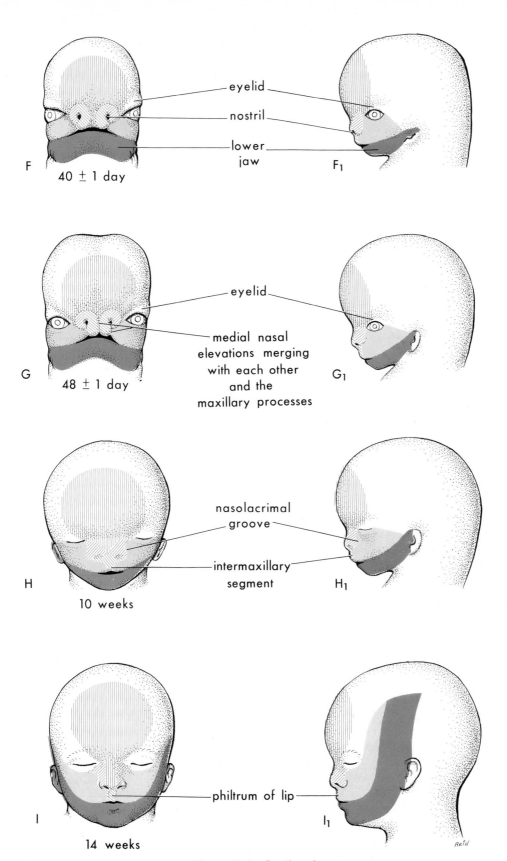

F   40 ± 1 day   F₁

- eyelid
- nostril
- lower jaw

G   48 ± 1 day   G₁

- eyelid
- medial nasal elevations merging with each other and the maxillary processes

H   10 weeks   H₁

- nasolacrimal groove
- intermaxillary segment

I   14 weeks   I₁

- philtrum of lip

Figure 11–9 *Continued.*

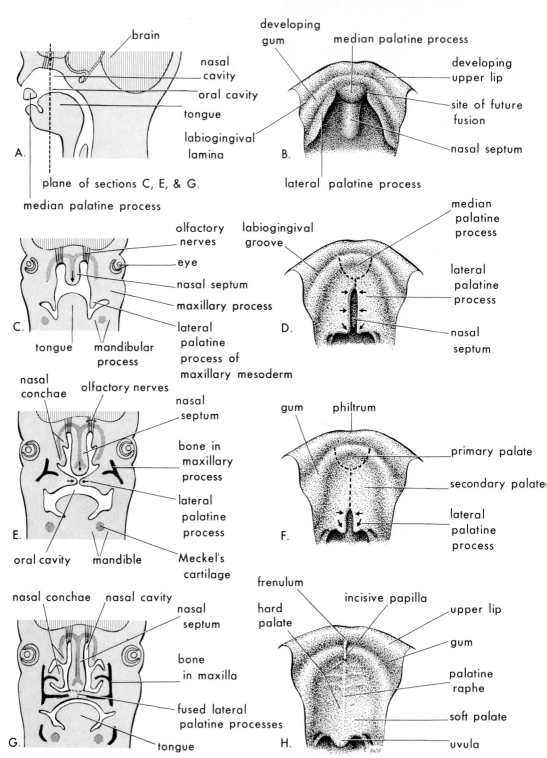

Figure 11–10. *A*, Sketch of a sagittal section of the embryonic head at the end of the sixth week showing the primary palate. *B, D, F* and *H*, Drawings of the roof of the mouth from the sixth to twelfth weeks illustrating development of the palate. The broken lines in *D* and *F* indicate sites of fusion of the palatine processes; the arrows indicate medial and posterior growth of the lateral palatine processes. *C, E,* and *G*, Drawings of frontal sections of the head illustrating fusion of the lateral palatine processes with each other and the nasal septum, and separation of the nasal and oral cavities.

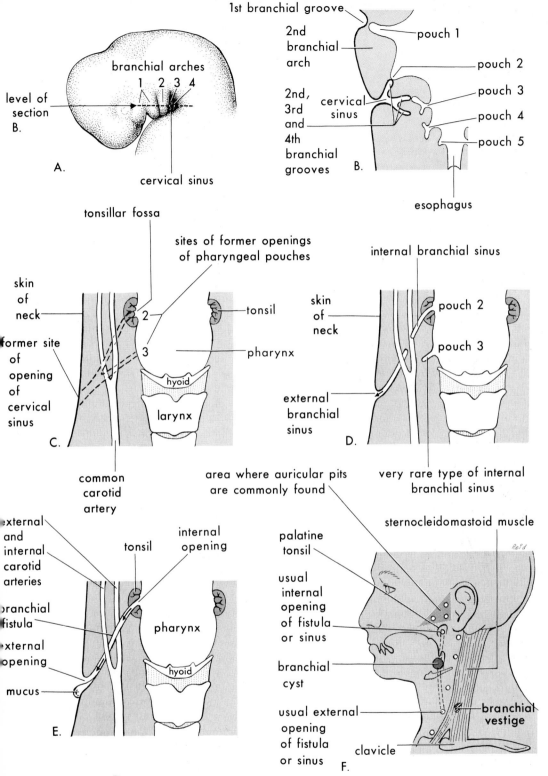

Figure 11–11. *A*, Drawing of the head and neck region of a five-week embryo. *B*, Horizontal section through the embryo, illustrating the relationship of the cervical sinus to the branchial arches and pharyngeal pouches. *C*, Diagrammatic sketch of the adult neck region, indicating the former sites of openings of the cervical sinus and the pharyngeal pouches. The broken lines indicate possible courses of branchial fistulas. *D*, Similar sketch showing the embryological basis of various types of branchial sinus. *E*, Drawing of a branchial fistula resulting from persistence of parts of the second branchial cleft and the second pharyngeal pouch. *F*, Sketch showing possible sites of branchial cysts and openings of branchial sinuses and fistulas. A branchial vestige is also illustrated.

to be remnants of the first branchial cleft, they probably represent ectodermal folds isolated during formation of the external ear.

Branchial or Lateral Cervical Sinus. Branchial sinuses are uncommon. They open externally on the side of the neck and result from failure of the second branchial cleft or groove to obliterate (Fig. 11–11C and D). Often there is an intermittent discharge of mucus from the opening.

Branchial sinuses which open into the pharynx are very rare. Because they usually open into the tonsillar fossa (Fig. 11–11D and F), these sinuses probably result from persistence of part of the second pharyngeal pouch.

Branchial Fistula. An abnormal tract opening both on the side of the neck and in the pharynx is called a branchial fistula (Fig. 11–11E and F). It usually results from persistence of parts of the second branchial groove and second pharyngeal pouch. The fistula ascends through the subcutaneous tissue and usually opens in the tonsillar fossa (Fig. 11–11E).

Branchial or Lateral Cervical Cyst. Remnants of parts of the cervical sinus, the second branchial groove or the second pharyngeal pouch may persist and form spherical or elongate cysts (Fig. 11–11F). Al-though they may be associated with branchial sinuses and drain through them, they often lie free in the neck just below the angle of the jaw.

The First Arch Syndrome. A pattern of multiple malformations resulting from abnormal transformation of first branchial arch components into various adult derivatives is often referred to as the first arch syndrome. The *Treacher-Collins syndrome* (mandibulofacial dysostosis) is characterized by malar hypoplasia with down-slanting palpebral fissures, defects of the lower lid, deformed external ear and sometimes abnormalities of the middle and inner ear. In the *Pierre Robin syndrome* (striking hypoplasia of the mandible), cleft palate and defects of the eye and ear are found.

Thyroglossal Duct Cysts and Duct Sinuses (Fig. 11–12). Cysts may form anywhere along the course followed by the thyroglossal duct during "descent" of the thyroid gland from the tongue. Normally, the thyroglossal duct atrophies and disappears, but remnants of it may persist and give rise to cysts in the tongue or in the midline of the neck, usually just below the hyoid bone. In about a third of cases, an opening through the skin exists as a result of perforation following infection of the cyst. This forms a thyroglossal duct sinus which usu-

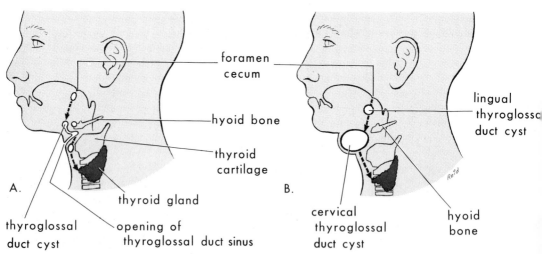

Figure 11–12. *A*, Diagrammatic sketch of the head, showing the possible locations of thyroglossal duct cysts. A thyroglossal duct sinus is also illustrated. The broken line indicates the course taken by the thyroglossal duct during descent of the thyroid gland from the foramen cecum to its final position in front of the trachea. *B*, A similar sketch illustrating lingual and cervical thyroglossal duct cysts. Most cysts are located near the hyoid bone.

ally opens in the midline of the neck anterior to the laryngeal cartilages.

Cleft Lip and Palate

Cleft lip and palate are common malformations of the face and palate. Although often associated, cleft lip and palate are embryologically and etiologically distinct malformations. They originate at different times during development and involve different developmental processes.

Cleft Lip (Fig. 11–13). This malformation of the upper lip, with or without cleft palate, occurs about once in 900 births; the defect may be unilateral or bilateral. The clefts vary from a small notch to a complete division of the lip and alveolar process.

Unilateral cleft lip results from failure of the maxillary process on the affected side to

merge with the merged medial nasal elevations.

Bilateral cleft lip results from failure of the maxillary processes to meet and merge with the medial nasal elevations. In complete bilateral cleft of the upper lip and alveolar process, the intermaxillary segment hangs free and projects anteriorly (Figs. 11–13C and D).

Cleft Palate (Figs. 11–14 and 11–15). Cleft palate, with or without cleft lip, occurs about once in 2500 births; the clefts may be unilateral or bilateral. A cleft may involve only the uvula, or it may extend through the soft and hard palates. In severe cases associated with cleft lip, the cleft in the anterior and posterior palate extends through the alveolar process and lip on both sides (Figs. 11–14G and H and 11–15B). The embryological basis of cleft palate is failure of the mesodermal masses of the lateral

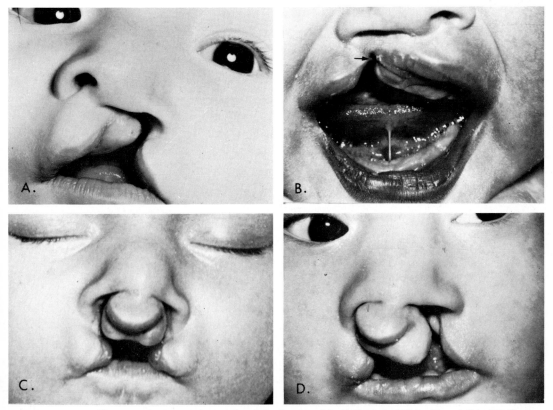

Figure 11–13. Photographs illustrating clefts of the lip. *A* and *B,* Unilateral cleft lip. The cleft in *B* is incomplete; the arrow indicates a band of tissue (Simonart's band) connecting the parts of the lip. *C* and *D,* Bilateral cleft lip. (Courtesy of Dr. D. A. Kernahan, The Children's Memorial Hospital, Chicago.)

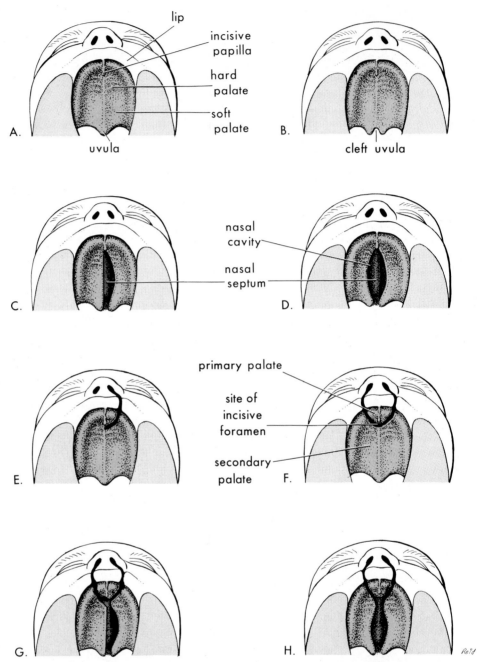

Figure 11–14. Drawings of various types of cleft lip and palate. *A*, Normal lip and palate. *B*, Cleft uvula. *C*, Unilateral cleft of the posterior or secondary palate. *D*, Bilateral cleft of the posterior palate. *E*, Complete unilateral cleft of the lip and alveolar process with a unilateral cleft of the anterior or primary palate. *F*, Complete bilateral cleft of the lip and alveolar process with bilateral cleft of the anterior palate. *G*, Complete bilateral cleft of the lip and alveolar process with bilateral cleft of the anterior palate and unilateral cleft of the posterior palate. *H*, Complete bilateral cleft of the lip and alveolar process with complete bilateral cleft of the anterior and posterior palate.

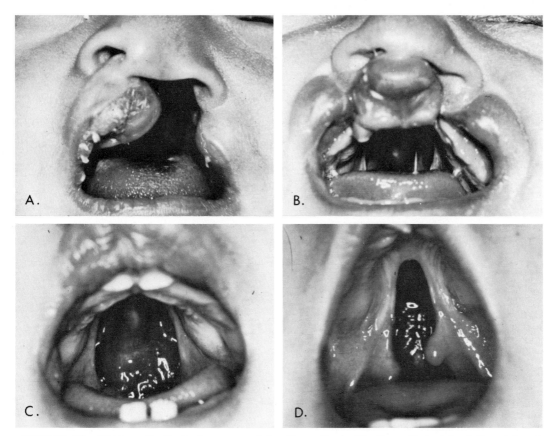

Figure 11–15. Photographs illustrating congenital malformations of the lip and/or palate. *A*, Complete unilateral cleft of the lip and alveolar process. *B*, Complete bilateral cleft of the lip and alveolar process with bilateral cleft of the anterior palate. *C* and *D*, Bilateral cleft of the posterior or secondary palate. The lip is normal. (Courtesy of Dr. Harry Medovy, Children's Centre, Winnipeg.)

palatine processes to meet and fuse with each other, with the nasal septum and/or with the median palatine process or primary palate.

Cleft lip and palate appear to have a mixed genetic and environmental causation. A sibling of a child with cleft palate has an elevated risk of having a cleft palate, but no increased risk of having a cleft lip.

Facial Clefts. Various types of facial cleft occur, but they are all extremely rare. Severe clefts are usually associated with gross malformations of the head. In *median cleft of the mandible* (Fig. 11–16*B*), there is a deep cleft resulting from failure of the mandibular processes of the first branchial arch to merge completely with each other.

Oblique facial clefts are often bilateral and extend from the upper lip to the medial margin of the orbit (Fig. 11–16*C*). They result from failure of the maxillary processes to merge with the lateral and medial nasal elevations. *Lateral* or *transverse facial clefts* run from the mouth toward the ear. Bilateral clefts leave the mouth very large, a condition called *macrostomia* (Fig. 10–16*D*); this abnormality results from failure of the maxillary and mandibular processes to merge.

Other Rare Facial Malformations. *Congenital microstomia* (small mouth) results from excessive merging of the maxillary and mandibular processes of the first arch (Fig. 11–16*E*). A *single nostril* results when only one nasal placode forms (Fig. 11–16*E*). *Bifid nose* results from failure of the medial nasal elevations to merge completely (Fig. 11–16*F*).

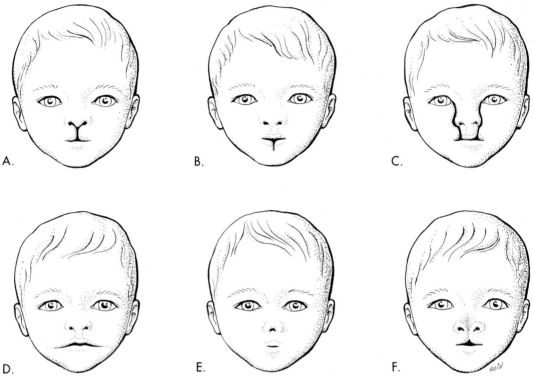

Figure 11–16. Drawings of very rare malformations of the face. *A,* Median cleft lip. *B,* Median cleft of the lower lip and jaw. *C,* Bilateral oblique facial clefts with complete bilateral cleft lip. *D,* Macrostomia or lateral facial cleft. *E,* Single nostril and microstomia; these malformations are not usually associated. *F,* Bifid nose and incomplete median cleft lip.

SUMMARY

During the fourth and fifth weeks, the primitive pharynx is bounded laterally by bar-like *branchial* or *pharyngeal arches.* Externally, between the arches, are branchial grooves. Internally, between the arches, are extensions of the pharynx called *pharyngeal pouches.* The arches, pouches and associated structures comprise the *branchial apparatus.*

Development of the tongue, face, lips, jaws, palate, pharynx and neck largely involves transformation of the branchial apparatus into adult structures. The branchial grooves disappear except for the first, which persists as the external acoustic meatus. The pharyngeal pouches give rise to the tympanic cavity and antrum, the pharyngotympanic tube, the palatine tonsil, the thymus and the parathyroid glands. The thyroid gland develops from a downgrowth from the floor of the pharynx in the region where the tongue develops.

Most congenital malformations of the head and neck originate during transformation of the branchial apparatus into adult structures. Branchial cysts, sinuses or fistulas may develop from parts of the second branchial groove or pharyngeal pouch which fail to obliterate. An ectopic thyroid gland results when the thyroid gland fails to descend, or only partially descends, from its site of origin in the tongue. The thyroglossal duct may persist or remnants of it may give rise to thyroglossal duct cysts; these cysts, if infected, may form thyroglossal duct sinuses which open in the midline of the neck.

Cleft lip is the most common congenital abnormality of the face. Although frequently associated with cleft palate, cleft lip and cleft palate are etiologically distinct malformations which involve different developmental processes occurring at different times. *Cleft lip* results from failure of mesodermal masses of the medial nasal elevations and maxillary processes to merge, whereas *cleft palate* results from failure of the mesodermal masses of the palatine processes to fuse.

12

THE RESPIRATORY SYSTEM

The *laryngotracheal groove* which appears during the fourth week in the caudal end of the primitive pharyngeal floor gives the first indication of the respiratory system (Fig. 12–1). Soon this groove deepens to form a diverticulum or outpouching ventral to the primitive pharynx (Fig. 12–2*A*). As this diverticulum grows caudally, it gradually separates from the pharynx. Tracheoesophageal folds grow toward each other and fuse to form the *tracheoesophageal septum* (Fig. 12–2*E*). This septum divides the cranial part of the foregut into the *laryngotracheal tube* and the *esophagus* (Fig. 12–2*F*).

THE LARYNX AND TRACHEA

The Larynx. The endodermal lining of the cranial end of the laryngotracheal tube and the surrounding mesenchyme develop into the larynx. The laryngeal cartilages develop from the branchial arch cartilages (see Chapter 11). The epiglottis develops from the caudal half of the *hypobranchial eminence* (Fig. 11–8). Folds of mucous membrane of the larynx become the *vocal folds (cords)*. The *laryngeal muscles* develop from muscle elements in the branchial arches.

The Trachea. The endodermal lining of

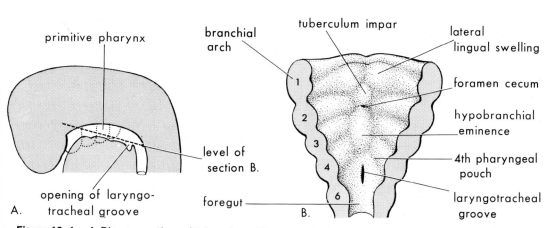

Figure 12–1. *A*, Diagrammatic sagittal section of the upper half of an embryo of about 26 days showing the laryngotracheal groove in the caudal end of the floor of the primitive pharynx (develops from the cranial part of the foregut). *B*, Horizontal section at the level shown in *A*, illustrating the floor of the primitive pharynx and the location of the laryngotracheal groove.

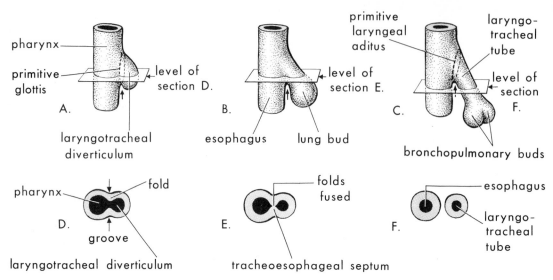

Figure 12–2. Successive stages of development of the tracheoesophageal septum during the fourth week. *A, B* and *C,* Lateral views of the caudal part of the primitive pharynx illustrating partitioning of the foregut into the esophagus and laryngotracheal tube. *D, E* and *F,* Transverse sections illustrating development of the tracheoesophageal septum and division of the cranial part of the foregut into the laryngotracheal tube and the esophagus.

the middle segment of the laryngotracheal tube gives rise to the epithelium and glands of the trachea. The cartilage, connective tissue and muscle of the trachea are derived from the surrounding splanchnic mesenchyme (Fig. 12–3).

THE BRONCHI AND LUNGS

A *lung bud* develops at the caudal end of the laryngotracheal tube (Fig. 12–4*A*) and soon divides into two *bronchopulmonary buds* (Fig. 12–4*B*). These buds differentiate into

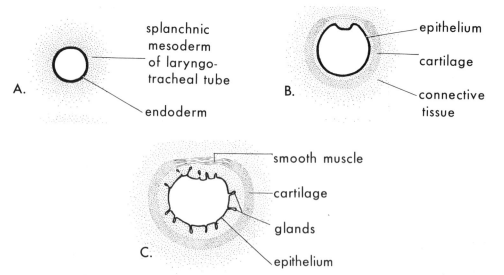

Figure 12–3. Drawings of transverse sections through the laryngotracheal tube illustrating progressive stages of development of the trachea. *A,* 4 weeks. *B,* 10 weeks. *C,* 11 weeks.

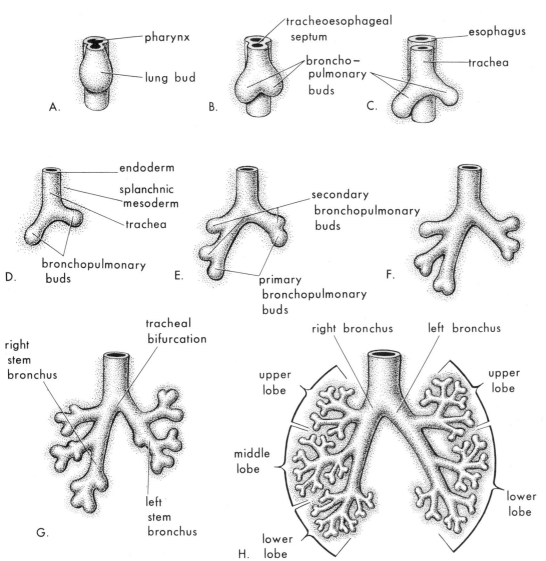

Figure 12–4. Drawings of ventral views illustrating successive stages in the development of the bronchi and lungs. *A to D*, 4 weeks. *E and F*, 5 weeks. *G*, 6 weeks. *H*, 8 weeks.

the bronchi and lungs and grow laterally into the *pericardioperitoneal canals* or *primitive pleural cavities* (Fig. 12–5*A*). Concurrently, the right bud gives rise to two secondary buds, whereas only one arises from the left bud (Fig. 12–4*E*). Subsequently, three lung lobes develop on the right side and two lobes form on the left (Fig. 12–4*H*). As the lungs develop, they acquire a layer of *visceral pleura* from the splanchnic mesoderm (Fig. 12–5). The thoracic body wall becomes lined by a layer of *parietal pleura*, derived from the somatic mesoderm. Lung development may be divided into four stages.

The Pseudoglandular Period (5 to 17 Weeks). Microscopically, the developing lung somewhat resembles a gland. The air-conducting system becomes established during this period.

The Canalicular Period (13 to 25 Weeks). The lumina of the bronchi and bronchioles enlarge, and the lung tissue becomes highly vascular. Each terminal bronchiole gives rise to two or more *respiratory bronchioles* (Fig. 12–6*A*). Each of these then divides into three to six sacculations called *alveolar ducts*. Toward the end of this period, the lining cells of these ducts become attenuated, per-

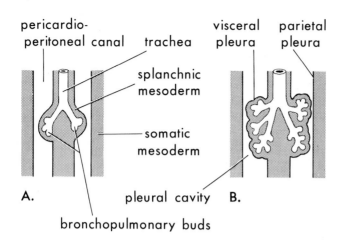

Figure 12–5. Diagrams illustrating the growth of the developing lungs into the splanchnic mesoderm of the medial walls of the pericardioperitoneal canals (primitive pleural cavities), and the development of the layers of the pleura. *A*, 5 weeks. *B*, 6 weeks.

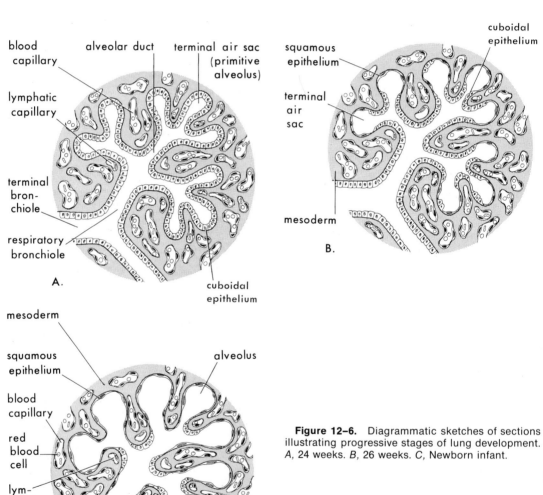

Figure 12–6. Diagrammatic sketches of sections illustrating progressive stages of lung development. *A*, 24 weeks. *B*, 26 weeks. *C*, Newborn infant.

mitting the blood capillaries to project as capillary loops into the future air spaces.

The Terminal Sac Period (24 Weeks to Birth). The alveolar ducts give rise to clusters of thin-walled terminal air sacs or primitive *pulmonary alveoli* (Fig. 12–6*A* and *B*). The capillary network proliferates rapidly in the mesenchyme around the developing alveoli, and there is concurrent active development of lymphatic capillaries. By 26 weeks, suf-

ficient terminal air sacs are usually present to permit survival of a prematurely born infant. The development of an adequate pulmonary vasculature is also critical to the survival of premature infants.

During this period the alveolar cells produce *surfactant*, a lipoprotein substance that covers the internal surface of the alveoli before birth. It is capable of lowering the surface tension at the air-alveolar interface, thereby maintaining patency of the alveoli and facilitating expansion of the lungs at birth. Absence or deficiency of surfactant appears to be a major cause of *hyaline membrane disease*, principally a disease of premature infants.

The Alveolar Period (Late Fetal Period to About Eight Years). The lining of the terminal air sacs becomes extremely thin, thus forming *characteristic pulmonary alveoli* (Fig. 12–6*C*). One-eighth to one-sixth of the adult number of alveoli are present at birth; their number increases until about the eighth year.

The lungs at birth are about half inflated with liquid derived from the lungs, the amniotic cavity and the tracheal glands. Consequently, aeration of the lungs at birth involves rapid replacement of intra-alveolar fluid by air.

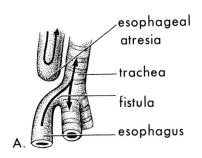

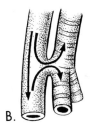

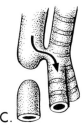

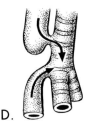

Figure 12–7. Sketches illustrating the four main varieties of tracheoesophageal fistula. Possible direction(s) of flow of contents is indicated by arrows. Esophageal atresia, as illustrated in *A*, occurs in about 90 per cent of cases.

esophageal atresia
trachea
fistula
esophagus

A.

B.

C.

D.

Congenital Malformations of the Lower Respiratory Tract

Tracheoesophageal Fistula. An abnormal passage or fistula connecting the trachea and esophagus occurs about once in every 2500 births. This condition results from incomplete division of the foregut into respiratory and digestive portions during the fourth and fifth weeks (Fig. 12–2). Incomplete fusion of the tracheoesophageal folds results in a defective tracheoesophageal septum and a communication between the trachea and the esophagus. There are four main varieties of tracheoesophageal fistula (Fig. 12–7). The most common is for the upper portion of the esophagus to end blindly (esophageal atresia) and for the lower portion to join the trachea near its bifurcation (Fig. 12–7*A*). As soon as the infant is fed, it chokes and becomes blue because the milk passes into the respiratory tract.

An excessive amount of amniotic fluid (polyhydramnios) is commonly associated with esophageal atresia and tracheoesophageal fistula because amniotic fluid cannot pass to the intestines for absorption and subsequent transfer to the placenta for disposal (see discussion of amniotic fluid in Chapter 8).

SUMMARY

The lower respiratory system begins to develop early in the fourth week from a median longitudinal *laryngotracheal groove* in the floor of the primitive pharynx. This groove deepens to produce a diverticulum which is soon separated from the foregut by the *tracheoesophageal septum.* The lining of the resulting laryngotracheal tube gives rise to the epithelium of the lower respiratory organs. The splanchnic mesenchyme surrounding this tube forms the connective tissue, cartilage, muscle, and blood and lymphatic vessels of these organs. The laryngotracheal tube divides at its termination into two *bronchopulmonary (lung) buds.* The one on the left divides into two buds and the one on the right into three buds; these develop into the adult lobes of the lung.

Lung development may be divided into four stages: (1) the *pseudoglandular period,* 5 to 17 weeks, when the bronchi and terminal bronchioles form; (2) the *canalicular period,* 13 to 25 weeks, when the lumina of the bronchi and terminal bronchioles enlarge, the respiratory bronchioles and alveolar ducts develop and the lung tissue becomes highly vascular; (3) the *terminal sac period,* 24 weeks to birth, when the alveolar ducts give rise to terminal air sacs (primitive alveoli); (4) the final stage of lung development is the *alveolar period,* late fetal period to about eight years of age, when the characteristic pulmonary alveoli develop.

Major congenital malformations of the lower respiratory system are rare, except for tracheoesophageal fistula. This common malformation results from faulty partitioning of the foregut into the esophagus and trachea.

13

THE DIGESTIVE SYSTEM

The primitive gut or digestive system forms during the fourth week, as the dorsal part of the yolk sac is enclosed in the embryo (Chapter 6). For descriptive purposes, the primitive gut is divided into three parts: the *foregut*, the *midgut* and the *hindgut*.

THE FOREGUT

The Esophagus.[1]   The partitioning of the trachea from the esophagus by the

---

[1]The foregut also gives rise to the lining epithelia and glands of the pharynx and lower respiratory system (see Chapters 11 and 12).

tracheoesophageal septum is described in Chapter 12. Initially the esophagus is very short (Fig. 13–1), but it soon reaches its final relative length. The smooth muscle of the esophagus develops from the surrounding splanchnic mesenchyme.

The Stomach.   The stomach first appears as a fusiform dilatation of the foregut (Figs. 13–1 and 13–2*A*); this primordium soon enlarges and broadens ventrodorsally (Fig. 13–2*B*). The dorsal border grows faster than the ventral border, producing the *greater curvature* (Fig. 13–2*C*). As the stomach acquires its adult shape, it rotates around its longitudinal axis.

Figure 13–1.   Drawing of a midsagittal section of a 4-week embryo showing the primitive gut or early digestive system and its blood supply.

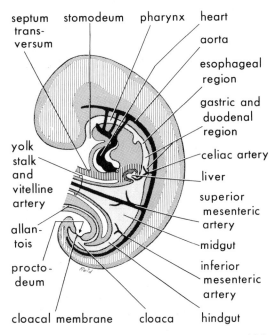

septum transversum   stomodeum   pharynx   heart
aorta
esophageal region
gastric and duodenal region
yolk stalk and vitelline artery
celiac artery
liver
superior mesenteric artery
allantois
midgut
proctodeum
inferior mesenteric artery
cloacal membrane   cloaca   hindgut

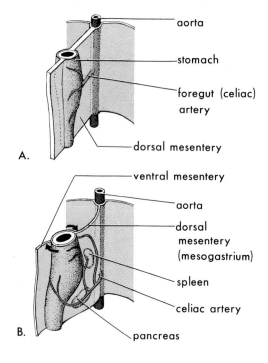

A.

- aorta
- stomach
- foregut (celiac) artery
- dorsal mesentery

B.

- ventral mesentery
- aorta
- dorsal mesentery (mesogastrium)
- spleen
- celiac artery
- pancreas

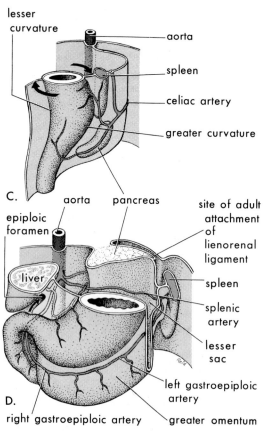

C.

- lesser curvature
- aorta
- spleen
- celiac artery
- greater curvature

D.

- epiploic foramen
- aorta
- pancreas
- site of adult attachment of lienorenal ligament
- spleen
- splenic artery
- lesser sac
- left gastroepiploic artery
- liver
- right gastroepiploic artery
- greater omentum

Figure 13–2. Drawings illustrating development and rotation of the stomach and formation of the greater omentum. *A,* About 30 days. *B,* About 35 days. *C,* About 40 days. *D,* About 48 days.

The stomach is suspended from the dorsal wall of the abdominal cavity by the dorsal *mesentery* or *dorsal mesogastrium* (Fig. 13–2*A*). The dorsal mesogastrium is carried to the left during rotation of the stomach and formation of a cavity known as the *lesser sac* (Fig. 13–2*A* to *C*). The lesser sac communicates with the main peritoneal cavity or *greater peritoneal sac* through a small opening, the *epiploic foramen* of Winslow (Fig. 13–2*D*).

The Duodenum. The duodenum develops from the caudal part of the foregut and the cranial part of the midgut. These parts grow rapidly and form a C-shaped loop that projects ventrally (Fig. 13–3*B* to *D*).

The Liver and Biliary Apparatus. The liver arises as a bud from the most caudal part of the foregut (Fig. 13–3*A*). This *hepatic diverticulum* extends into the *septum transversum*, where it rapidly enlarges and divides into two parts:

1. The large cranial part is the primordium of the liver. As the endodermal liver cords develop and penetrate the septum transversum, they break up the umbilical and vitelline veins forming the *hepatic sinusoids*. The fibrous and *hemopoietic tissue* and *Kupffer cells* of the liver are derived from the splanchnic mesenchyme of the septum transversum. The liver grows rapidly and soon fills most of the abdominal cavity (see Fig. 6–10*C* and *D*). *Hemopoiesis* (formation and development of blood cells) begins during the sixth week; this activity is mainly responsible for the relatively large size of the liver during the second month. By nine weeks, the liver represents about 10 per cent of the total weight of the fetus.

2. The small caudal portion of the hepatic diverticulum expands to form the *gall bladder* (Fig. 13–3*C*). The stalk connecting the hepatic and cystic ducts to the duodenum becomes the common *bile duct*.

The Pancreas. The pancreas develops from *dorsal and ventral pancreatic buds* of endodermal cells that arise from the caudal part of the foregut (Fig. 13–4*A*). When the duodenum grows and rotates to the right (clockwise), the ventral bud is carried dorsally and fuses with the dorsal bud (Fig. 13–4*D* and *G*).[2]

---

[2]The spleen (part of the lymphatic system) is derived from a mass of mesenchymal cells between the layers of the dorsal mesogastrium (Fig. 13–4*D*). The spleen acquires its characteristic shape early in the fetal period.

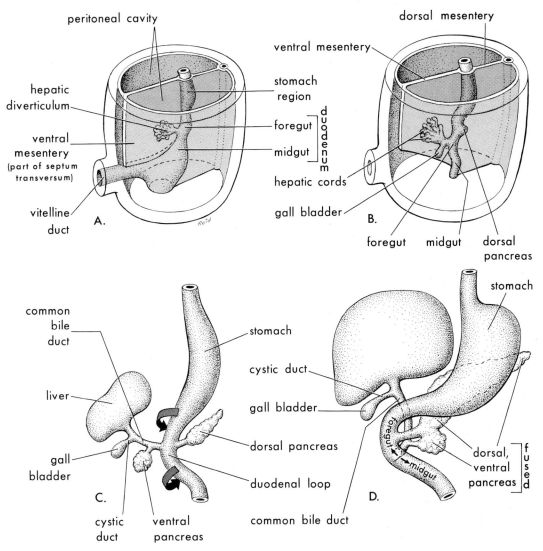

Figure 13-3. Drawings illustrating progressive stages in the development of the duodenum, liver, pancreas and extrahepatic biliary apparatus. *A*, 4 weeks. *B* and *C*, 5 weeks. *D*, 6 weeks.

THE MIDGUT

Rotation and Fixation of the Midgut. At first the midgut communicates widely with the yolk sac (Fig. 13–1), but this connection soon becomes reduced to the narrow *yolk stalk* or vitelline duct (Fig. 13–5*A*).

Herniation of the midgut. As the midgut elongates, it forms a ventral U-shaped *midgut loop* which projects into the umbilical cord (Fig. 13–5*A*). This "herniation" is a normal migration of the midgut into the extraembryonic coelom which occurs because there is not enough room in the abdomen. The space shortage is caused mainly by the relatively massive liver and kidneys. Within the umbilical cord, the *midgut loop rotates counterclockwise*, as viewed from the ventral aspect of the embryo (Fig. 13–5*B*), around the axis of the *superior mesenteric artery*. This brings the proximal limb of the midgut loop to the right and the distal limb to the left (Fig. 13–5*B* and *B₁*).

Return of the midgut. During the tenth week, the intestines return rapidly to the abdomen; the so-called "reduction of the midgut hernia." As the intestines return, they undergo further rotation (Fig. 13–5*C₁* and *D₁*). The decrease in the relative size of the liver and kidneys and enlargement of

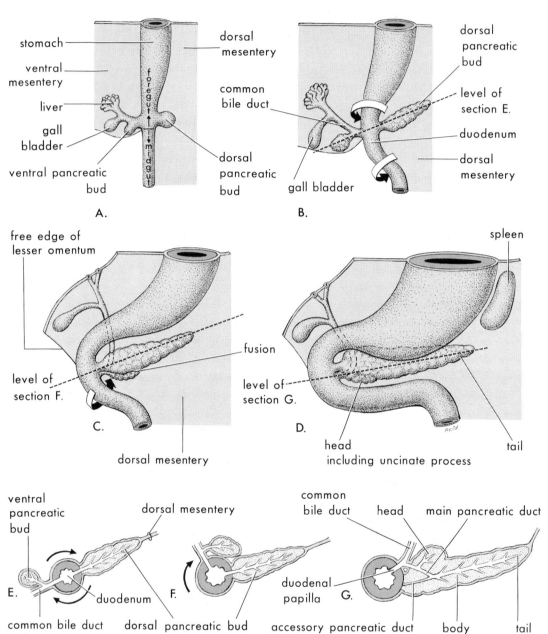

Figure 13–4. *A* to *D*, Schematic drawings showing the successive stages in the development of the pancreas from the fifth to the seventh weeks. *E* to *G*, Diagrammatic transverse sections through the duodenum and the developing pancreas. Growth and rotation (arrows) of the duodenum bring the ventral pancreatic bud toward the dorsal bud, and they subsequently fuse. Note that the common bile duct initially attaches to the ventral aspect of the duodenum, and is carried around to the dorsal aspect as the duodenum rotates.

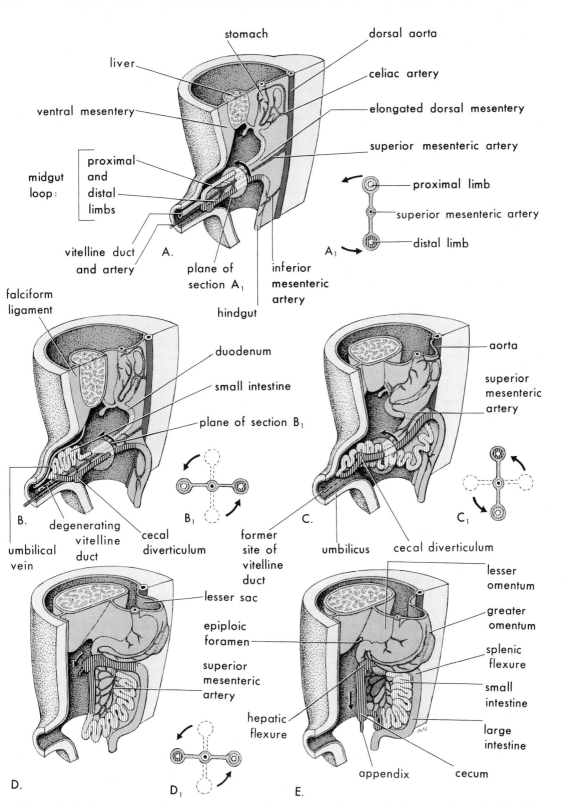

Figure 13–5. Drawings showing rotation of the midgut, as seen from the left. *A*, Around the end of the fifth week, showing the midgut loop partially within the umbilical cord. Note the elongated, double-layered dorsal mesentery containing the superior mesenteric artery. *A₁*, Transverse section through the midgut loop illustrates the initial relationship of the limbs of the midgut to the artery. *B*, Later stage showing the beginning of the midgut rotation. *B₁* illustrates the 90° counterclockwise rotation which carries the proximal limb to the right. *C*, About 10 weeks, showing the intestines returning to the abdomen. *C₁* illustrates a further rotation of 90°. *D*, Slightly later, following return of intestines to the abdomen. *D₁* shows there has been a further 90° rotation of the gut, making a total of 270°. *E*, Late fetal period, after descent of the cecum to its normal position and fixation of the gut.

the abdominal cavity are likely important factors related to the return of the intestines to the abdomen.

Fixation of the midgut. Lengthening of the proximal part of the colon gives rise to the hepatic flexure and ascending colon (Fig. 13–5D and E). This results in the cecum and appendix "descending" from the upper to the lower right quadrant of the abdomen. As the intestines assume their final positions, their mesenteries are pressed against the posterior wall of the abdominal cavity. The mesentery of the ascending colon gradually disappears. The other derivatives of the midgut loop retain their mesenteries.

The Cecum and Appendix. The primordium of the cecum and appendix is the *cecal diverticulum* which appears during the fifth week. This conical pouch appears on the caudal limb of the midgut loop (Fig. 13–5B). The distal end or apex of this blind sac does not grow so rapidly, and thus the appendix forms (Fig. 13–5E). By birth it is a long blind tube, relatively longer than in the adult.

THE HINDGUT

The hindgut extends from the midgut to the cloacal membrane. This membrane is composed of endoderm of the cloaca and ectoderm of the proctodeum or *anal pit* (Fig. 13–6). The expanded terminal part of the hindgut, the *cloaca* receives the allantois ventrally.

The cloaca is divided by a coronal sheet of mesenchyme, the *urorectal septum*, which develops in the angle between the allantois and the hindgut (Fig. 13–6B). As this septum grows toward the cloacal membrane, infoldings of the lateral walls of the cloaca form (Fig. 13–6B₁). These folds grow toward each other and fuse, dividing the cloaca into two parts: (1) the *rectum and upper anal canal* dorsally, and (2) the *urogenital sinus* ventrally (Fig. 13–6D and F). By the end of the sixth week, the urorectal septum has fused with the cloacal membrane, dividing it into a dorsal *anal membrane* and a larger ventral *urogenital membrane* (Fig. 13–6E and F). These membranes rupture at the end of the seventh week, thus establishing the *anal canal.*

CONGENITAL MALFORMATIONS OF THE DIGESTIVE SYSTEM

Esophageal Atresia (Fig. 12–7A). Esophageal atresia often occurs with tracheoesophageal fistula (see Chapter 12), but it may occur as a separate malformation. Atresia or stenosis usually results from abnormal division of the foregut into respiratory and digestive portions.

Pyloric Stenosis. The lumen of the pylorus is reduced, principally because the sphincteric muscle layer is hypertrophied. This common abnormality affects one in about 200 newborn males and one in 1000 newborn females. The cause of the condition is unknown.

Malformations of the Intestines

Omphalocele or Exomphalos (Fig. 13–7). This condition occurs once in about 6600 births and results from failure of the intestines to return to the abdomen at the end of the first stage of rotation of the midgut loop. The hernia may consist of a single loop of bowel or it may contain most of the intestines and also include the liver, spleen and pancreas. The covering of the hernial sac is the amnion of the umbilical cord.

Nonrotation (Fig. 13–8A). This relatively common condition, often called "left-sided colon," is often asymptomatic, but volvulus (twisting) of the intestines may occur. In non-rotation, the midgut loop does not complete the final 180 degrees of rotation; thus the small intestine lies on the right side of the abdomen and the entire large intestine on the left.

Mixed Rotation and Volvulus (Fig. 13–8B). The cecum lies below the pylorus and is fixed to the posterior abdominal wall by peritoneal bands which pass over the duodenum. These bands and the frequent presence of a volvulus of the intestines usually cause duodenal obstruction. This type of malrotation results from failure of the midgut loop to complete its rotation.

Reversed Rotation (Fig. 13–8C). Rarely, the intestines rotate in a clockwise rather than counterclockwise direction. Thus the duodenum lies anterior to the transverse colon. As a result, the transverse colon may be obstructed.

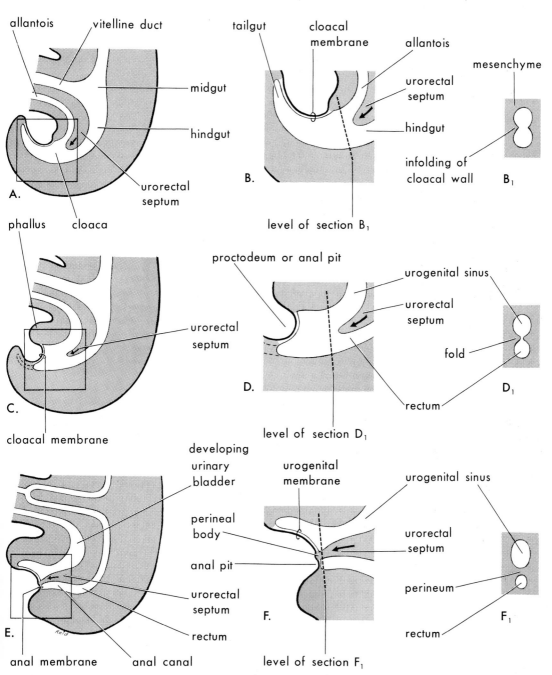

Figure 13–6. Drawings illustrating successive stages in the partitioning of the cloaca into the rectum and urogenital sinus by the urorectal septum. *A, C* and *E,* Views from the left side at 4, 6 and 7 weeks, respectively. *B, D* and *F* are enlargements of the cloacal region. *B₁, D₁* and *F₁* are transverse sections through the cloaca at the levels shown in *B, D* and *F.*

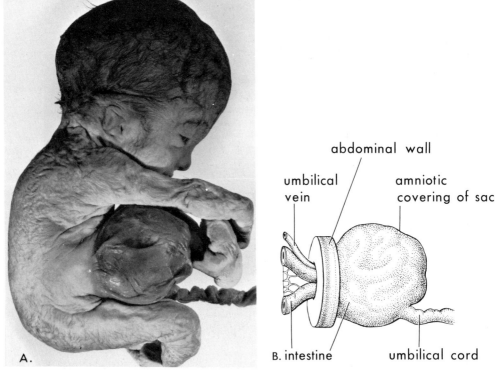

Figure 13-7. *A*, Large omphalocele in a 28-week fetus. *Half actual size. B*, Drawing illustrating the structure and contents of the hernial sac.

Subhepatic Cecum (Fig. 13-8*D*). Failure of the proximal part of the colon to elongate occurs in about six per cent of fetuses, and results in the adult cecum and appendix being located below the liver.

Mobile Cecum. About 10 per cent of persons have this condition, which results from incomplete fixation of the ascending colon. It is significant because of the possible variations in position of the appendix and because volvulus of the cecum may occur.

Paraduodenal or Internal Hernia (Fig. 13-8*E*). During return of the midgut to the abdomen, the small intestine passes into the mesentery of the midgut loop, forming a hernia-like sac. This uncommon condition rarely produces symptoms.

Midgut Volvulus (Fig. 13-8*F*). Because the mesenteries fail to undergo normal fixation, twisting of the intestines commonly occurs with malrotation of the midgut loop. The small intestine hangs by a narrow stalk formed by the superior mesenteric vessels, and they usually twist around this stalk and cause duodenal obstruction,

Intestinal Stenosis and Atresia. Narrowing or stenosis (Fig. 13-9*A*) and complete obstruction or atresia of the intestinal lumen (Fig. 13-9*B*) occur most often in the duodenum and ileum. Failure of an adequate number of vacuoles to form during intestinal recanalization leaves a transverse diaphragm, a so-called *diaphragmatic atresia* (Fig. 13-9*F$_2$*). Failure of an adequate number of vacuoles to form during recanalization, or perforation of a transverse diaphragm, can also produce stenosis (Fig. 13-9*E$_2$*).

Meckel's Diverticulum and Other Yolk Sac Remnants. A Meckel's diverticulum of the ileum is one of the commonest malformations of the digestive tract, and is of clinical significance because it sometimes becomes inflamed and causes symptoms mimicking appendicitis. The wall of the diverticulum contains all layers of the ileum and may contain gastric and pancreatic tissues. The gastric mucosa often secretes acid, producing ulceration (Fig. 13-10*A*). A Meckel's diverticulum occurs in two to four per cent of

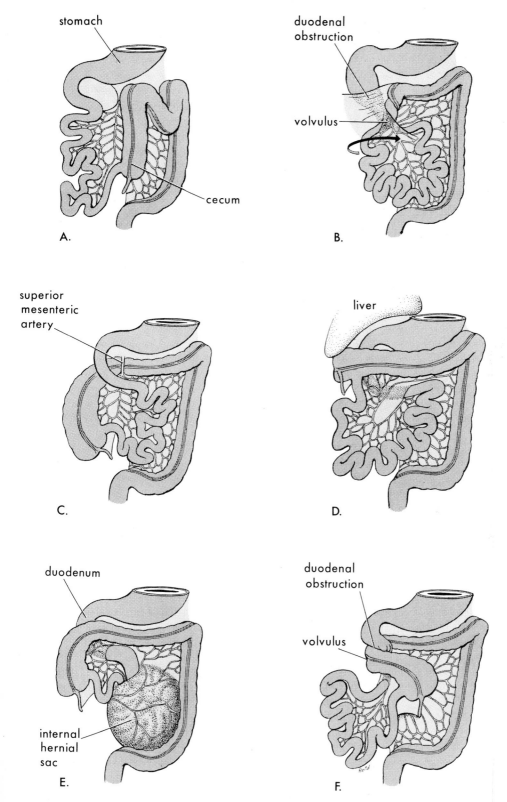

Figure 13–8. Drawings illustrating various abnormalities of midgut rotation. *A*, Nonrotation. *B*, Mixed rotation and volvulus (twisting of the intestines). *C*, Reversed rotation. *D*, Subhepatic cecum. *E*, Paraduodenal hernia. *F*, Midgut volvulus.

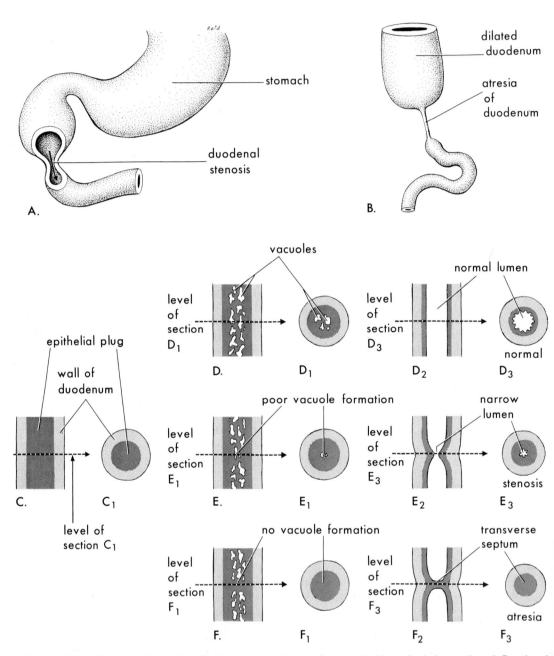

Figure 13–9. Diagrams illustrating the two common types of congenital intestinal obstruction. *A*, Duodenal stenosis. *B*, Duodenal atresia. *C* to *F*, Diagrammatic longitudinal and transverse sections of the duodenum showing: (1) normal recanalization (*D* to D_3), (2) stenosis (*E* to E_3) and (3) atresia (*F* to F_3).

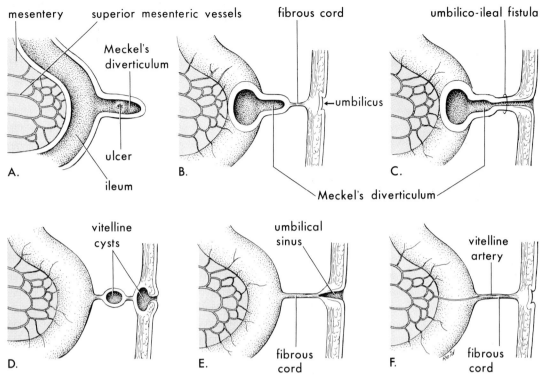

Figure 13-10. Drawings illustrating Meckel's diverticulum and other remnants of the yolk stalk. *A*, Section of the ileum and a Meckel's diverticulum with ulcer. *B*, A Meckel's diverticulum connected to the umbilicus by a fibrous cord. *C*, Umbilico-ileal fistula resulting from persistence of the entire intra-abdominal portion of the yolk stalk. *D*, Vitelline cysts at the umbilicus and in a fibrous remnant of the yolk stalk. *E*, Umbilical sinus resulting from the persistence of the yolk stalk near the umbilicus. The sinus is not always connected to the ileum by a fibrous cord as illustrated. *F*, The yolk stalk has persisted as a fibrous cord connecting the ileum with the umbilicus. A persistent vitelline artery extends along the fibrous cord to the umbilicus.

persons and is the remnant of the *yolk stalk.* Typically, it appears as a finger-like pouch, about three to six cm long.

Imperforate Anus and Related Malformations

Some form of imperforate anus occurs once in about 5000 births. Most anorectal malformations result from abnormal development of the urorectal septum, resulting in incomplete separation of the cloaca into urogenital and anorectal portions (Fig. 13–6). If the urorectal septum fails to develop, a *persistent cloaca* results (Fig. 13–11*A*).

Anal Agenesis With or Without Fistula (Fig. 13–11*D* and *E*). The anal canal may end blindly, but more often there is an abnormal opening (ectopic anus) or fistula which opens into the perineum. The fistula may, however, open into the vulva in females or into the urethra in males. Anal agenesis with fistula results from incomplete separation of the cloaca by the urorectal septum.

Anal Stenosis (Fig. 13–11*B*). The anus is in the normal position, but the anal canal is narrow. This malformation probably results from a slight dorsal deviation of the urorectal septum as it grows caudally to fuse with the cloacal membrane.

Membranous Atresia of the Anus (Fig. 13–11*C*). The anus is in the normal position, but a thin layer of tissue separates the anal canal from the exterior. This rare condition results from failure of the anal membrane to perforate at the end of the seventh week.

Anorectal Agenesis With or Without Fistula (Fig. 13–11*F* and *G*). The rectum ends

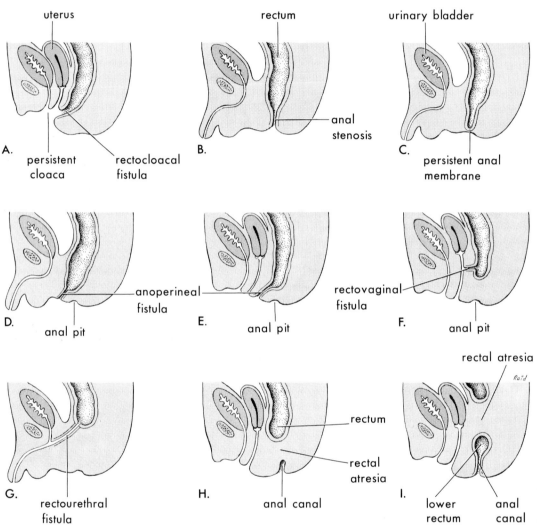

Figure 13–11. Drawings illustrating various anorectal malformations. *A*, Persistent cloaca. Note the common outlet for the intestinal, urinary and reproductive tracts. This very rare condition usually occurs in females. *B*, Anal stenosis. *C*, Membranous atresia (covered anus). *D* and *E*, Anal agenesis with fistula. *F*, Anorectal agenesis with rectovaginal fistula. *G*, Anorectal agenesis with rectourethral fistula. *F* and *G* are sometimes called persistent cloaca. *H* and *I*, Rectal atresia.

well above the anal canal; *this is the most common type of anorectal malformation.* Although the rectum may end blindly, there is usually a fistula to the urethra in males or to the vagina in females. Anorectal agenesis has an embryological basis similar to anal agenesis described previously.

Rectal Atresia (Fig. 13–11*H* and *I*). Both the anal canal and rectum are present, but they are separated by an atretic (blocked) segment of rectum. The cause of rectal atresia may be abnormal recanalization or defective blood supply, as discussed with malformations of the small intestines.

SUMMARY

The *primitive gut* forms during the fourth week by incorporation of the roof of the yolk sac into the embryo. It consists of three parts. The *foregut* gives rise to the pharynx and lower respiratory system, the esophagus, the stomach, the duodenum (as far as the common bile duct), the liver, the pancreas and the biliary apparatus.

The *midgut* gives rise to the duodenum (distal to the common bile duct), the jejunum, the ileum, the cecum, the appendix, the ascending colon and the right or proximal half to two-thirds of the transverse colon. The midgut herniates into the umbilical cord during the fifth week because of inadequate room in the abdomen. During the tenth week, the intestines rapidly return to the abdomen. Omphalocele, malrotation and abnormalities of fixation result from failure of or abnormal return of the intestines to the abdomen. Because the gut is normally occluded at one stage, stenosis (narrowing), atresia (obstruction) and duplications may result if recanalization fails to occur or occurs abnormally. Various remnants of the yolk stalk may persist; *Meckel's diverticulum* is common and is clinically significant.

The *hindgut* gives rise to the left or distal one-third to half of the transverse colon, the descending and sigmoid (pelvic) colon, the rectum and the upper part of the anal canal. The remainder of the anal canal develops from the anal pit or proctodeum. The caudal part of the hindgut is expanded into the *cloaca*, which is divided by the *urorectal septum* into the urogenital sinus and rectum. At first, the rectum is separated from the exterior by the *anal membrane*, but this normally breaks down at the end of the seventh week. Most anorectal malformations arise from abnormal partitioning of the cloaca by the urorectal septum into anorectal and urogenital parts.

14

THE UROGENITAL SYSTEM

Development of the urinary (excretory) and genital (reproductive) systems is closely associated and parts of one system are used by the other and vice versa. Development of the urogenital system is easier to understand if the urinary and genital systems are described separately.

THE URINARY OR EXCRETORY SYSTEM

The Kidney and Ureter

Three successive sets of excretory organs develop in human embryos: the *pronephros*, the *mesonephros* and the *metanephros*. The third set remains as the permanent kidneys.

The pronephros (or "forekidney") is a transitory, nonfunctional structure which appears early in the fourth week (Fig. 14–1*A*). The pronephros soon degenerates, but most of its duct is utilized by the next kidney (Fig. 14–1*B*).

The mesonephros (or "midkidney") appears later in the fourth week caudal to the rudimentary pronephros (Fig. 14–1). It may function while the permanent kidney is developing. By the end of the embryonic period, the mesonephros has degenerated and disappeared, except for its duct and a few tubules which persist as genital ducts in males or form vestigial remnants in females.

The metanephros (or "hindkidney") is the one which becomes the *permanent kidney*. It

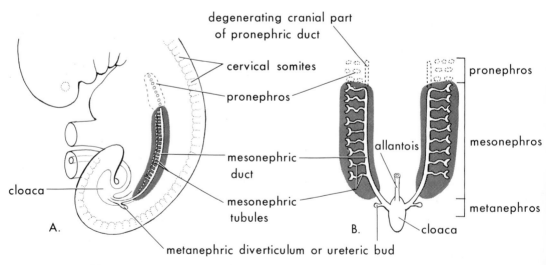

Figure 14–1. Diagrammatic sketches illustrating the three sets of excretory structures present in an embryo of about 29 days. *A*, Lateral view. *B*, Ventral view. The metanephros becomes the permanent kidney.

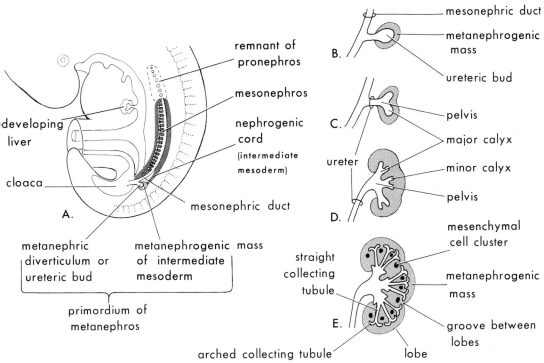

Figure 14–2. *A,* Sketch of a lateral view of a five-week embryo showing the primordium of the metanephros or permanent kidney. *B* to *E,* Sketches showing successive stages of development of the ureteric bud (fifth to eighth weeks) into the ureter, pelvis, calyces and collecting tubules. The renal lobes illustrated in *E* are visible in the kidneys of newborn infants. The external evidence of the lobes normally disappears by the end of the first year.

appears in the fifth week and begins to function about three weeks later. Urine formation continues actively throughout fetal life. The urine mixes with the amniotic fluid which the fetus drinks (see Chapter 8).

The metanephros develops from two sources: the *metanephric diverticulum,* or ureteric bud, and the *metanephrogenic mass* of mesoderm (Fig. 14–2*A* and *B*). The metanephric diverticulum is a dorsal bud from the mesonephric duct which grows into the metanephrogenic mass of mesoderm (Fig. 14–2*B*). The stalk of the ureteric bud becomes the ureter, and its expanded cranial end forms the renal pelvis. The pelvis divides into *major* and *minor calyces,* from which collecting tubules soon grow (Fig. 14–2*C* to *E*). Each collecting tubule undergoes repeated branching, forming successive generations of collecting tubules. Near the blind end of each arched collecting tubule (Fig. 14–3*A*), clusters of mesenchymal cells develop into metanephric tubules (Fig. 14–3*B*). The ends of these tubules are invaginated by an ingrowth of the fine blood vessels, the *glomerulus,* to form a double-layered cup, the glomerular (Bowman's) capsule.

The renal corpuscle (glomerulus and capsule) and its associated tubules form a *nephron.* The distal convoluted tubule of the nephron contacts an arched collecting tubule, and the two tubules soon become confluent.

Positional Changes of the Kidney (Fig. 14–4). Initially, the kidneys are in the pelvis, but they gradually come to lie in the abdomen. As the kidneys move out of the pelvis, they are supplied by arteries at successively higher levels. The caudal arteries normally degenerate as the kidney ascends and new vessels form.

The Bladder and Urethra

Division of the cloaca by the *urorectal septum* into a dorsal rectum and a ventral urogenital sinus is described in Chapter 13, and is illustrated in Figure 14–5*A, C, E,* and *G.* The urinary bladder and urethra are derived from the urogenital sinus and from the adjacent splanchnic mesenchyme. As the bladder enlarges, the caudal portions of the mesonephric ducts are incorporated

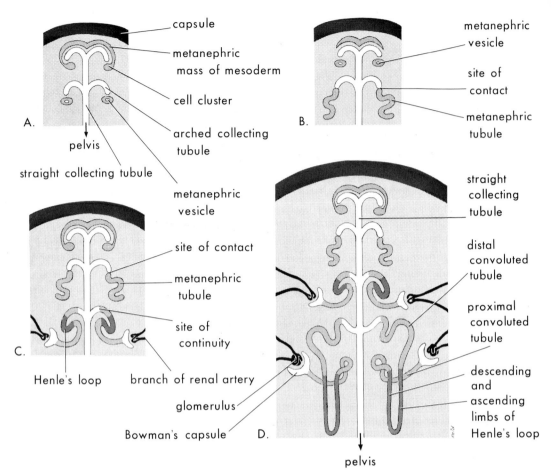

Figure 14–3. Diagrammatic sketches illustrating stages in the development of nephrons. The nephrons become continuous with the collecting tubules to form uriniferous tubules.

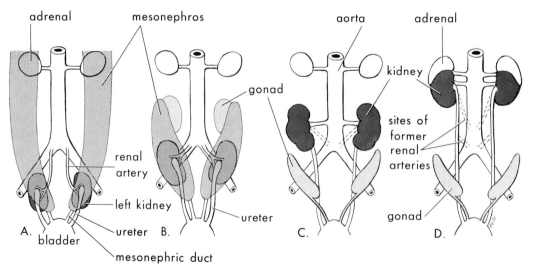

Figure 14–4. Diagrams of ventral views of the abdominopelvic region of embryos and fetuses (sixth to ninth weeks) showing the medial rotation and ascent of the kidneys from the pelvis to the abdomen. Note that as the kidneys ascend, they are supplied by arteries at successively higher levels.

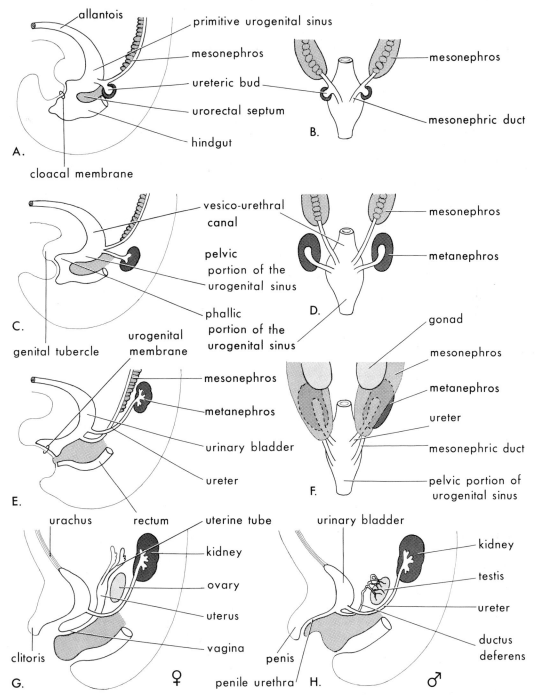

Figure 14–5. Diagrams showing (1) division of the cloaca into the urogenital sinus and the rectum, (2) absorption of the mesonephric ducts, (3) development of the urinary bladder, urethra and urachus and (4) changes in the location of the ureters. *A,* Lateral view of the caudal half of a five-week embryo. *B, D* and *F,* dorsal views. *C, E, G* and *H,* lateral views. The stages shown in *G* and *H* are reached by about 12 weeks.

into its dorsal wall (Fig. 14–5). As the mesonephric ducts are absorbed, the ureters come to open separately into the urinary bladder (Fig. 14–5C to F).

The Adrenal or Suprarenal Gland

The cortex and medulla of the adrenal glands have different origins. The *cortex* develops from mesoderm and the medulla from neuroectoderm. The cells which form the medulla are derived from the neural crest which appears as the neural tube forms (see Chapter 17). The cells which form the *adrenal cortex* are derived from the epithelium lining the posterior abdominal wall. During the fifth week, cells migrate from adjacent sympathetic ganglia and form a cellular mass on the medial side of the fetal cortex (Fig. 14–6C). These cells are gradually encapsulated by the fetal cortex as they differentiate into the *chromaffin cells* of the adrenal (suprarenal) medulla (Fig. 14–6D). Differentiation of the characteristic adrenal cortical zones begins during the late fetal period, but is not complete until the end of the third year.

THE GENITAL OR REPRODUCTIVE SYSTEM

Although the genetic sex of an embryo is determined at fertilization by the kind of sperm that fertilizes the ovum (see Chapter 3), there is no real indication of sex until the seventh week, when the *gonads* (future ovaries or testes) begin to acquire sexual characteristics. The early genital system is similar in both sexes, and initially all normal human embryos are potentially bisexual. This period of early genital development is referred to as the *indifferent stage* of the reproductive organs.

Development of Testes and Ovaries

The Indifferent Gonads (Fig. 14–6). Gonadal development is first indicated during the fifth week, when a thickened area of epithelium, the *"germinal" epithelium*, develops on the medial aspect of the urogenital ridge (Fig. 14–6C). Proliferation of cells soon produces a bulge on the medial side of

each mesonephros known as the *gonadal ridge*. Finger-like epithelial cords, called *primary sex cords*, soon grow into the underlying mesenchyme (Fig. 14–6D). The indifferent gonad now consists of an outer *cortex* and an inner *medulla*. In embryos with an XX sex chromosome complex (complement), the cortex normally differentiates into an ovary, and the medulla regresses. In embryos with an XY sex chromosome complex, the medulla normally differentiates into a testis, and the cortex regresses.

Large spherical primitive sex cells, called *primordial germ cells*, are visible early in the fourth week on the wall of the yolk sac. These cells later migrate along the dorsal mesentery of the hindgut to the gonadal ridges (Fig. 14–6), and become incorporated in the primary sex cords.

Sex Determination. Genetic sex is established at fertilization. Gonadal sex is determined by the sex chromosome complex. The Y chromosome has a strong testis-determining effect on the medulla of the indifferent gonad. Under its influence, the primary sex cords differentiate into seminiferous tubules (Fig. 14–7B and D). Absence of a Y chromosome results in formation of an ovary (Fig. 14–7C and E). Thus, the type of sex chromosome complex established at fertilization determines the type of gonad that develops from the indifferent gonad.

Development of Testes (Fig. 14–7B, D and F). In embryos with a Y chromosome, the primary sex cords condense and branch; their ends anastomose to form the *rete testis*. The prominent sex cords, now called *seminiferous* or *testicular* cords, lose their connections with the germinal epithelium as the thick fibrous capsule called the *tunica albuginea* develops (Fig. 14–7B and D). The seminiferous cords develop into the *seminiferous tubules*, the *tubuli recti* and the *rete testis*. The walls of the seminiferous tubules are composed of two kinds of cells (Fig. 14–7F): supporting or *sustentacular cells of Sertoli*, derived from the germinal epithelium, and *spermatogonia*, derived from the primordial germ cells.

Development of Ovaries (Figs. 14–7C, E and G). In embryos lacking a Y chromosome, gonadal development occurs very slowly. The ovary is not identifiable until about the tenth week. Thereafter the characteristic cortex begins to develop. The pri-

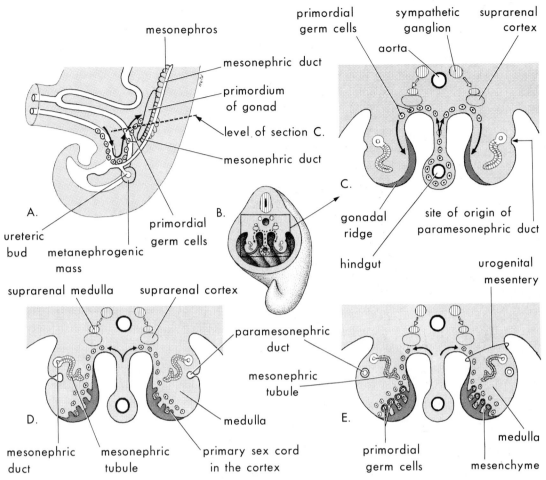

Figure 14–6. *A*, Sketch of five-week embryo illustrating the migration of primordial germ cells. *B*, Three-dimensional sketch of the caudal region of a five-week embryo showing the location and extent of the gonadal ridges on the medial aspect of the urogenital ridges. *C*, Transverse section showing the primordium of the adrenal glands, the gonadal ridges and the migration of primordial germ cells. *D*, Transverse section through a six-week embryo showing the primary sex cords and the developing paramesonephric ducts. *E*, Similar section at later stage showing the indifferent gonads and the mesonephric and paramesonephric ducts.

mary sex cords do not become prominent in the gonads of female embryos. They form a rudimentary rete ovarii which soon disappears.

During the fetal period, *cortical cords* extend from the germinal epithelium into the underlying mesenchyme (Fig. 14–7C). As these cords increase in size, primordial germ cells are incorporated into them. The cords break up into isolated cell clusters called *primordial follicles*, consisting of an *oogonium* derived from a primordial germ cell surrounded by a layer of follicular cells (Fig. 14–7E and G). Active mitosis of oogonia occurs during fetal life, producing thousands of these primitive germ cells. *No oogonia form postnatally in full-term humans.*

Development of the Genital Ducts

The Indifferent Stage (Fig. 14–8). Two pairs of genital ducts develop in both sexes: *mesonephric ducts* and *paramesonephric ducts* (Fig. 14–6D). The paramesonephric ducts come together in the midline and fuse into a Y-shaped *uterovaginal primordium* or canal (Fig. 14–8A). The funnel-shaped openings of the ducts open into the coelomic or peritoneal cavity. The uterovaginal primordium

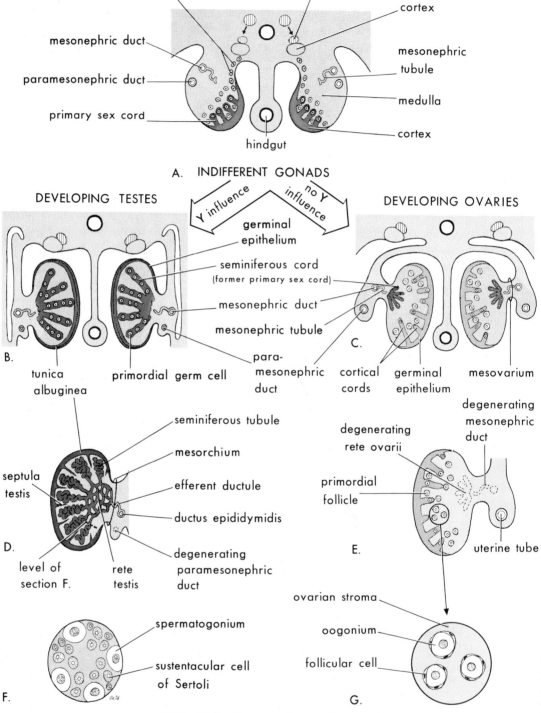

primordial germ cells   suprarenal medulla   suprarenal cortex

mesonephric duct

paramesonephric duct

primary sex cord

mesonephric tubule

medulla

cortex

hindgut

A.   INDIFFERENT GONADS

DEVELOPING TESTES

Y influence   no Y influence

DEVELOPING OVARIES

germinal epithelium

seminiferous cord
(former primary sex cord)

mesonephric duct

mesonephric tubule

para-mesonephric duct

B.

tunica albuginea   primordial germ cell

C.

cortical cords   germinal epithelium   mesovarium

seminiferous tubule

mesorchium

efferent ductule

ductus epididymidis

degenerating paramesonephric duct

septula testis

D.

level of section F.   rete testis

degenerating rete ovarii

primordial follicle

degenerating mesonephric duct

uterine tube

E.

ovarian stroma

oogonium

follicular cell

spermatogonium

sustentacular cell of Sertoli

F.

G.

Figure 14–7. *See opposite page for legend.*

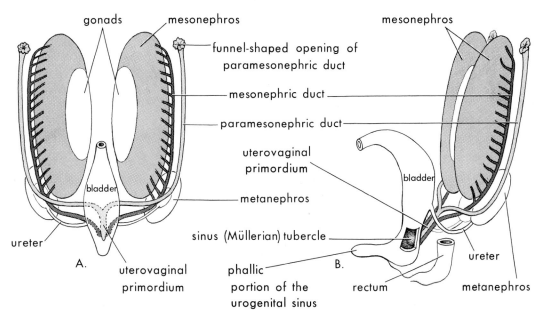

Figure 14–8. *A,* Sketch of a frontal view of the posterior abdominal wall of a seven-week embryo showing the two pairs of genital ducts present during the indifferent stage. *B,* Lateral view of a nine-week fetus showing the sinus (Müllerian) tubercle on the posterior wall of the urogenital sinus.

projects into the dorsal wall of the urogenital sinus and produces an elevation, called the *sinus* or *Müllerian tubercle* (Fig. 14–8*B*).

The fetal testes produce at least two hormones: one stimulates development of the mesonephric ducts into the male genital tract; the other suppresses development of the paramesonephric ducts into female ducts.

Development of the Male Genital Ducts. When the mesonephros degenerates, some mesonephric tubules near the testis persist and are transformed into *efferent ductules* or *ductuli efferentes* (Fig. 14–9*A*). These ductules open into the mesonephric duct which be-

comes the *ductus epididymidis* in this region. Beyond the epididymis, the mesonephric duct acquires a thick investment of smooth muscle and becomes the *ductus deferens.* A lateral outgrowth from the caudal end of each mesonephric duct gives rise to a *seminal vesicle.* The part of the mesonephric duct between the duct of this gland and the urethra becomes the *ejaculatory duct.* The remainder of the male genital duct system consists of the urethra.

The Prostate Gland. Multiple endodermal outgrowths arise from the prostatic portion of the urethra and grow into the surrounding mesenchyme. The glandular

Figure 14–7. Schematic sections illustrating the differentiation of the indifferent gonads into testes or ovaries. *A,* Six weeks, showing the indifferent gonads composed of an outer cortex and an inner medulla. *B,* Seven weeks, showing testes developing under the influence of a Y chromosome. Note that the primary sex cords have become seminiferous cords and that they are separated from the germinal epithelium by the tunica albuginea. *C,* 12 weeks, showing ovaries beginning to develop. Cortical (secondary sex) cords have extended from the germinal epithelium, displacing the primary sex cords centrally into the mesovarium, where they form the rudimentary rete ovarii. *D,* Testis at 20 weeks, showing the rete testis and the seminiferous tubules derived from the seminiferous cords. An efferent ductule has developed from a mesonephric tubule, and the mesonephric duct has become the ductus epididymidis. *E,* Ovary at 20 weeks, showing the primordial follicles formed from the cortical cords. The rete ovarii derived from the primary sex cords and the mesonephric tubule and duct are regressing. *F,* Section of a seminiferous tubule from a 20-week fetus. Note that no lumen is present at this stage and that the seminiferous epithelium is composed of two kinds of cells. *G,* Section from the ovarian cortex of a 20-week fetus showing three primordial follicles.

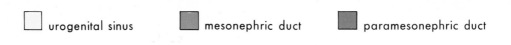

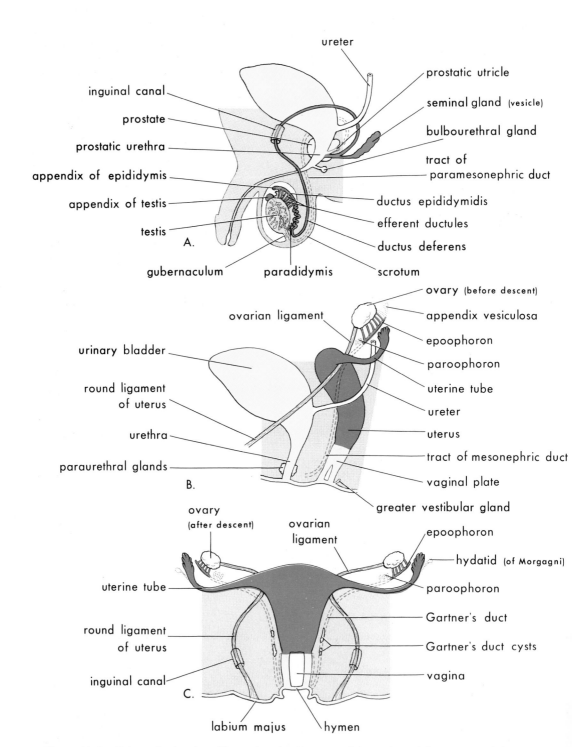

Figure 14–9. Schematic drawings illustrating development of the male and female reproductive systems from the primitive genital ducts. Vestigial structures (paradidymis, paroophoron, appendix of testis, appendix of epididymis, Gartner's duct, hydatid of Morgagni) are also shown. For more information about these, see Moore (1973). *A,* Reproductive system in a newborn male. *B,* Female reproductive system in a 12-week fetus. *C,* Reproductive system in a newborn female.

epithelium of the prostate differentiates from these endodermal cells, and the associated mesenchyme differentiates into the stroma and smooth muscle fibers of the prostate.

The Bulbourethral Glands (Cowper's Glands). These pea-sized structures develop from paired endodermal outgrowths from the membranous portion of the urethra. The smooth muscle fibers and the stroma differentiate from the adjacent mesenchyme.

Development of the Female Genital Ducts. In female embryos, the mesonephric ducts regress and the paramesonephric ducts develop into the female genital tract. The cranial unfused portions of the paramesonephric ducts develop into the uterine tubes, and the fused portions, or *uterovaginal primordium*, give rise to the epithelium and glands of the uterus (Fig. 14–9B and C). The endometrial stroma and the myometrium are derived from the adjacent mesenchyme.

Development of the Vagina. The vaginal epithelium is derived from the endoderm of the urogenital sinus, and the fibromuscular wall of the vagina develops from the uterovaginal primordium. A solid cord of endodermal cells called the vaginal plate forms, the central cells of which later break down and form the lumen of the vagina. The peripheral cells remain as the vaginal epithelium (Fig. 14–9C). Until late fetal life, the lumen of the vagina is separated from the cavity of the urogenital sinus by a membrane called the *hymen* (Figs. 14–9C and 14–10H). The hymen usually ruptures during the perinatal period.

Auxiliary Genital Glands. Buds grow out from the urethra into the surrounding mesenchyme and form the *urethral glands* and the paraurethral glands (of Skene). These glands correspond to the prostate gland in the male. Similar outgrowths from the urogenital sinus form the greater vestibular glands (of Bartholin), which are homologous with the bulbourethral glands in the male.

Descent of the Testes. Inguinal canals develop and later form pathways for the testes to descend through the abdominal wall into the scrotum. Inguinal canals develop in female embryos even though the ovaries do not enter the inguinal canals. Descent of the testes through the inguinal canals usually begins during the twenty-eighth week and takes about three days. About four weeks later, the testes enter the scrotum and the inguinal canals contract. The descent of the testis explains why the ductus deferens crosses anterior to the ureter (Fig. 14–9A).

Development of the External Genitalia

The Indifferent Stage (Fig. 14–10A and B). The external genitalia also pass through a stage that is not distinguishable as male or female. Early in the fourth week, a *genital tubercle* develops ventral to the cloacal membrane, and *labioscrotal swellings* and *urogenital folds* develop on each side of the cloacal membrane. The genital tubercle soon elongates and is called a *phallus;* initially it is as large in females as in males (Fig. 14–10C and D). A *urethral groove* forms on the ventral (under) surface of the phallus. Although external sexual characteristics begin to appear during the early fetal period (Fig. 14–10C and D), the external genitalia of males and females appear somewhat similar until the end of the ninth week. The final form is not established until the twelfth week (Fig. 14–10G and H).

Development of Male External Genitalia (Fig. 14–10C, E and G). Masculinization of the indifferent external genitalia is caused by androgens produced by the fetal testes. As the phallus elongates to form the *penis,* the *urogenital folds* fuse with each other along the ventral (under) surface of the penis from behind forward to form the *penile urethra.* As a result, the external urethral orifice moves progressively toward the *glans penis* (Fig. 14–10 C and E).

Development of Female External Genitalia (Fig. 14–10D, F and H). Feminization of the indifferent external genitalia occurs in the absence of androgens. The phallus becomes the relatively small *clitoris;* it develops like the penis except that the urogenital folds do not fuse. The unfused urogenital folds form the *labia minora.* The labioscrotal folds largely remain unfused and form the *labia majora.*

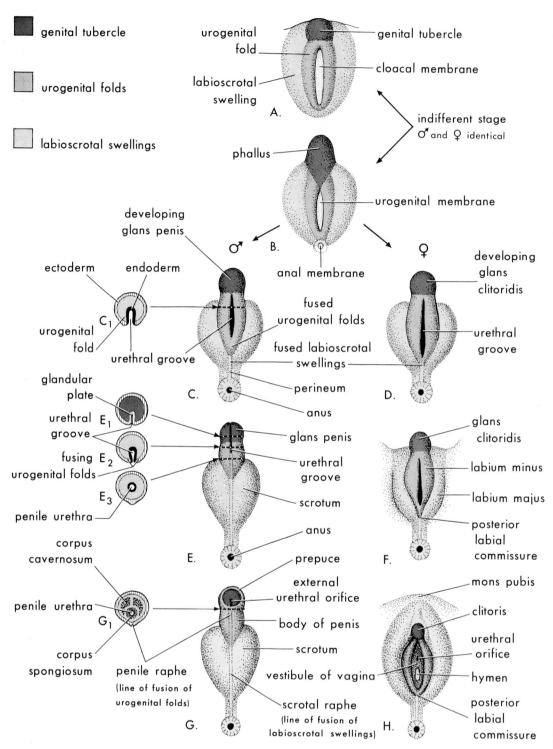

Figure 14–10. *A* and *B*, Diagrams illustrating development of the external genitalia during the indifferent stage (four to seven weeks). *C, E* and *G*, Stages in the development of male external genitalia at about 9, 11 and 12 weeks, respectively. To the left are schematic transverse sections (C_1, E_1 to E_3 and G_1) through the developing penis illustrating formation of the penile urethra. *D, F* and *H*, Stages in the development of female external genitalia at 9, 11 and 12 weeks, respectively.

CONGENITAL MALFORMATIONS OF THE UROGENITAL SYSTEM

Abnormalities of the kidney and ureter occur in three to four per cent of the population and include variations in blood supply, abnormal positions and duplications.

Duplications of the Upper Urinary Tract (Fig. 14–11*B*, *C* and *F*). Duplications of the ureter and pelvis are relatively common, but a supernumerary kidney is rare. These abnormalities result from division of the metanephric diverticulum or ureteric bud. Formation of two ureteric buds or division of a ureteric bud results in a supernumerary kidney if the divided portions of the bud are widely separated.

Renal Agenesis (Fig. 14–11*A*). Unilateral absence of a kidney is relatively common. Renal agenesis probably results from failure of a ureteric bud to develop.

Simple Renal Ectopia (Fig. 14–11*B*). One or both kidneys may be in an abnormal position. *Pelvic kidney* results from failure of the kidney to ascend. Pelvic kidneys may fuse to form a round mass known as a *discoid* or *pancake kidney* (Fig. 14–11*E*).

Crossed Renal Ectopia (Fig. 14–11*D*). During ascent, a kidney may cross to the opposite side and fuse with the other kidney, producing a single large kidney.

Horseshoe Kidney (Fig. 14–12). The kidneys are fused across the midline in one in about 600 persons. The large U-shaped kidney usually lies at the level of the lower lumbar vertebrae and generally produces no symptoms.

Exstrophy of the Bladder (Fig. 14–13). Protrusion of the posterior wall of the urinary bladder occurs in this uncommon congenital abnormality. Exstrophy of the bladder results from failure of mesenchymal cells to migrate between the surface ectoderm and the urogenital sinus during the fourth week. Thus, no muscle forms in the portion of the anterior abdominal wall over the urinary bladder. Later this thin wall ruptures and the posterior wall of the bladder protrudes.

Intersexuality

Because an early embryo has the potential to develop into a male or female, errors in sex development result in various degrees of intermediate sex, a condition known as *intersexuality* or *hermaphroditism*. A person with ambiguous external genitalia is called a hermaphrodite. Intersexual conditions are classified according to the histological appearance of the gonads. All *true hermaphrodites* have both ovarian and testicular tissue. Some *pseudohermaphrodites* have testes and are called male pseudohermaphrodites; others have ovaries and are known as female pseudohermaphrodites. Fortunately, intersexuality is uncommon.

True Hermaphrodites. Persons with this extremely rare condition usually have a 46, XX chromosome constitution. Both ovarian and testicular tissue are present, either in the same or in opposite gonads. The physical appearance may be male or female but the external genitalia are usually ambiguous. This condition results from an error in sex determination.

Male Pseudohermaphrodites. These persons have a 46, XY chromosome constitution. The external and internal genitalia are intersexual and variable, resulting from varying degrees of development of the phallus and paramesonephric ducts. Either an inadequate amount of androgenic hormones is produced, or they are formed after the period of maximum tissue sensitivity of the sexual structures has passed.

Testicular Feminization (Fig. 14–14). Persons with this rare condition (related to intersexuality) appear as normal females despite the presence of testes and XY sex chromosomes. Normal breast development occurs at puberty. The vagina ends blindly and the other internal genitalia are absent or rudimentary. The testes are usually intra-abdominal or inguinal, but they may descend into the labia majora. Embryologically, these females represent an extreme form of male pseudohermaphroditism, but they are not intersexes in the usual sense because they have normal feminine external genitalia. Although testes develop and secrete androgens, masculinization of the genitalia fails to occur apparently because the indifferent external genitalia were insensitive to androgens.

Female Pseudohermaphrodites. These persons have a 46, XX chromosome constitution. The most common cause of female pseudohermaphroditism is the *adrenogenital syndrome*, resulting from congenital virilizing adrenal hyperplasia (Fig. 14–15). There is

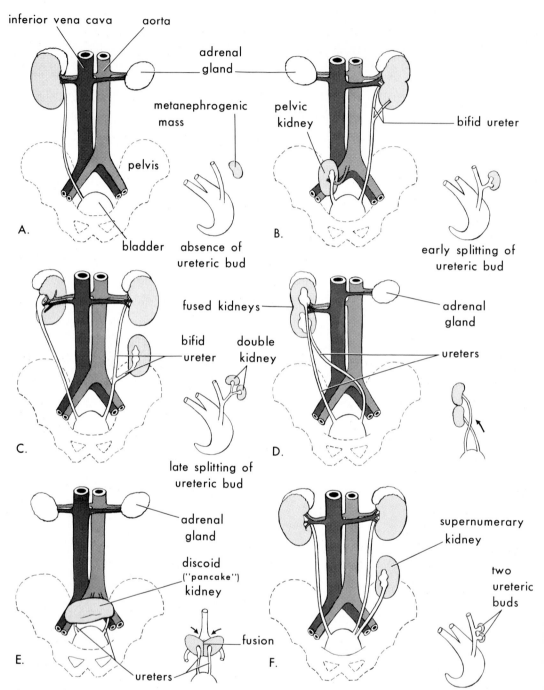

Figure 14–11. Drawings illustrating various abnormalities of the upper urinary tract. The small sketch to the lower right of each drawing illustrates the probable embryological basis of the malformation. *A,* Unilateral renal agenesis. *B,* Right side, pelvic kidney; left side, bifid ureter. *C,* Right side, malrotation of the kidney; left side, bifid ureter and two kidneys. *D,* Crossed renal ectopia. The left kidney crossed to the right side and fused with the right kidney. *E,* "Pancake" or discoid kidney resulting from fusion of the unascended kidneys. *F,* Supernumerary left kidney resulting from the development of two ureteric buds.

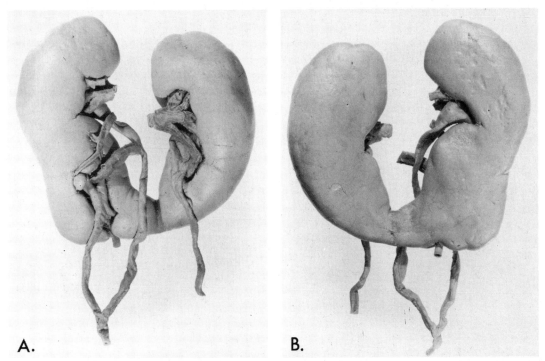

Figure 14–12. Photographs of a horseshoe kidney resulting from fusion of the lower poles of the kidneys. *A*, Anterior view. *B*, Posterior view. *Half actual size.* The larger right kidney has a bifid ureter.

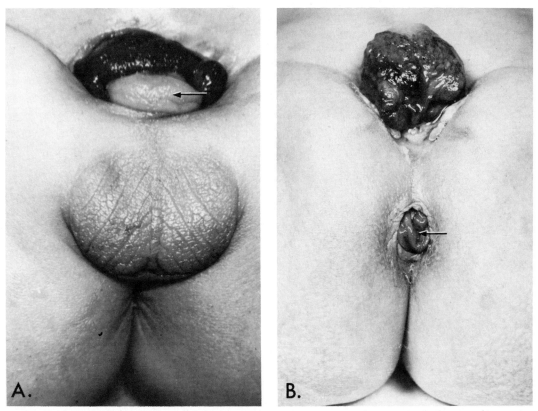

Figure 14–13. Photographs of infants with exstrophy of the bladder. *A*, Male. Epispadias is also present and the penis (arrow) is small. (Courtesy of Dr. Colin C. Ferguson, Children's Centre of Winnipeg.) *B*, Female. The arrow indicates a slight prolapse of the rectum. (Courtesy of Mr. Innes Williams, Genitourinary Surgeon, The Hospital for Sick Children, Great Ormond Street, London, England.)

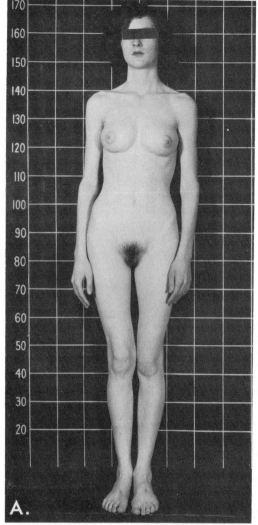

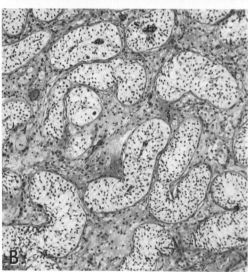

no ovarian abnormality, but the excessive production of androgens by the fetal adrenal glands causes masculinization of the external genitalia, varying from enlargement of the clitoris to almost masculine genitalia. Commonly, there is clitoral hypertrophy and partial fusion of the labia majora (Fig. 14–15). Persons with this syndrome are the most frequently encountered group of intersexes, accounting for about half of all cases of ambiguous external genitalia. *Prompt recognition and treatment of the associated adrenal imbalance are most important.* Congenital virilizing adrenal hyperplasia is caused by recessive mutant genes.

Female pseudohermaphrodites who do not have congenital virilizing adrenal hyperplasia are very rare. The administration of certain hormones to a mother during pregnancy may cause similar abnormalities of the fetal external genitalia (see Fig. 9–12).

Hypospadias (Fig. 14–16*A* to *C*). Once in about every 300 males, the external urethral orifice is on the ventral (under) surface of the penis instead of at the tip of the glans. Usually the penis is curved downward or ventrally, a condition known as *chordee.* There are four types of hypospadias: *glandular, penile, penoscrotal* and *perineal.* The glandular and penile types constitute about 80 per cent of cases. Hypospadias results from an inadequate production of androgens by the fetal testes; this causes failure of fusion of the urogenital folds. Differences in the timing and degree of hormonal failure account for the variety of types of hypospadias.

Epispadias (Fig. 14–16*D*). Once in about every 30,000 infants, the urethra opens on the dorsal (upper) surface of the penis. Although epispadias may occur as a separate entity, it is often associated with exstrophy of the bladder (Fig. 14–13) and has a similar cause.

Cryptorchidism or Undescended Testes. This condition occurs in about three per

Figure 14–14. *A,* Photograph of a 17-year-old female with the syndrome of testicular feminization. *B,* Photomicrograph of a section through a testis removed from the inguinal region of this girl showing seminiferous tubules. There are no germ cells. (From Jones, H. W., and Scott, W. W.: *Hermaphroditism, Genital Anomalies and Related Endocrine Disorders.* 1958. Courtesy of the Williams & Wilkins Co.)

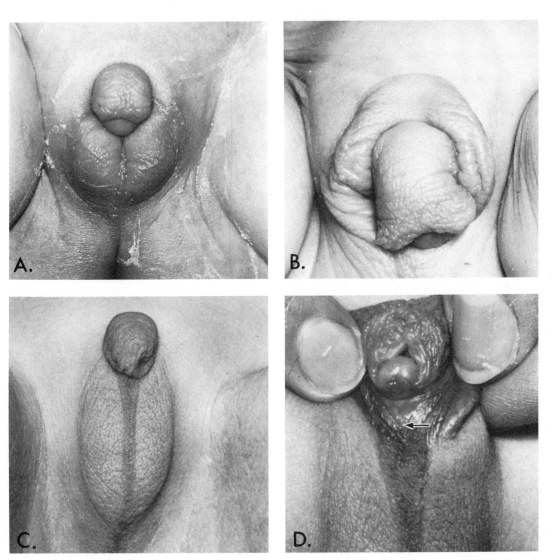

Figure 14–15. Photographs of the external genitalia of female pseudohermaphrodites resulting from congenital virilizing adrenal hyperplasia. *A,* External genitalia of a newborn female, exhibiting enlargement of the clitoris and fusion of the labia majora. *B,* External genitalia of a female infant, showing considerable enlargement of the clitoris. The labia majora have partially fused to form a scrotum-like structure. *C* and *D,* External genitalia of this six-year-old girl showing the enlarged clitoris and fused labia majora. In *D,* note the glans clitoridis and the opening of the urogenital sinus (arrow).

cent of male infants. A cryptorchid testis may be located in the abdominal cavity or anywhere along the usual path of descent of the testis; usually it lies in the inguinal canal. The cause of most cases of cryptorchidism is unknown, but failure of normal androgen production appears to be a factor.

Uterovaginal Malformations (Fig. 14–17). Various types of uterine duplication result from failure of the paramesonephric ducts to fuse normally during formation of the uterus. Double uterus results from failure of fusion of the lower parts of the paramesonephric ducts and may be associated with a double or a single vagina (Fig. 14–17*A* and *B*). If the doubling involves only the upper portion of the body of the uterus, the condition is called *bicornuate (double-horn) uterus* (Fig. 14–17*C* and *D*). In some cases, the uterus is divided internally by a thin septum (Fig. 14–17*F*). Very rarely, one paramesonephric duct degenerates or fails

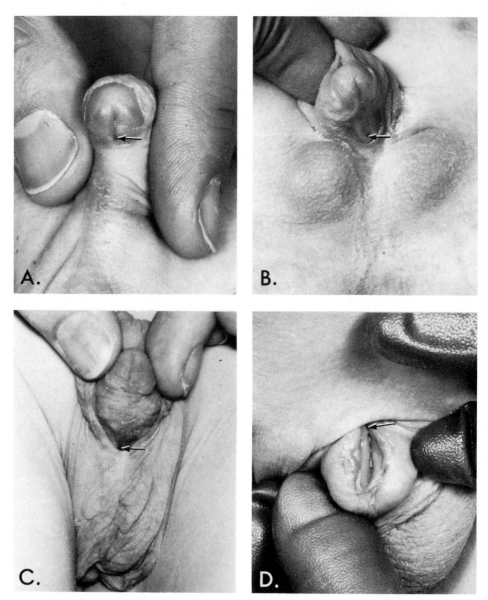

Figure 14–16. Photographs of penile malformations. *A,* Glandular hypospadias. The external urethral orifice is indicated by the arrow. There is a shallow pit at the usual site of the orifice. There is a moderate degree of chordee causing the penis to curve ventrally. (From Jolly, H.: *Diseases of Children,* 2nd Ed. 1968. Courtesy of Blackwell Scientific Publications.) *B,* Penile hypospadias. The penis is short and curved (chordee). The external urethral orifice (arrow) is near the penoscrotal junction. *C,* Penoscrotal hypospadias. The external urethral orifice (arrow) is located at the penoscrotal junction. *D,* Epispadias. The external urethral orifice (arrow) is on the dorsal (upper) surface of the penis near its origin. (Courtesy of Mr. Innes Williams, Genitourinary Surgeon, The Hospital for Sick Children, Great Ormond Street, London, England.)

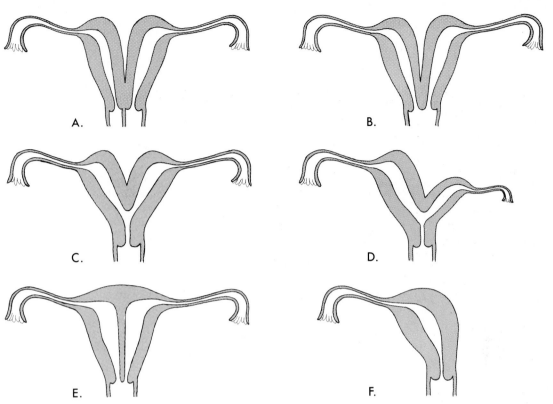

Figure 14–17. Drawings illustrating various types of congenital uterine abnormalities. *A,* Double uterus (uterus didelphys) and double vagina. *B,* Double uterus with single vagina. *C,* Bicornuate uterus. *D,* Bicornuate uterus with a rudimentary left horn. *E,* Septate uterus. *F,* Unicornuate uterus.

to form; this results in a *unicornuate (single horn) uterus* (Fig. 14–17*F*).

Once in about every 4000 females *absence of the vagina* occurs. This results from failure of the vaginal plate to develop. When the vagina is absent, the uterus is usually also absent. Failure of canalization of the vaginal plate results in *vaginal atresia.* Failure of the hymen to rupture results in a condition known as *imperforate hymen.*

SUMMARY

Three successive sets of kidneys develop: (1) the transitory vestigial and nonfunctional *pronephros,* (2) the *mesonephros,* which may serve as a temporary excretory organ, and (3) the functional *metanephros* or permanent kidney.

The metanephros develops from two sources: (1) the metanephric diverticulum or ureteric bud, which gives rise to the ureter, the renal pelvis, the calyces and the collecting tubules, and (2) the metanephric mass of mesoderm, which gives rise to the nephrons. At first the kidneys are located in the pelvis, but they gradually ascend to the abdomen. The urinary bladder develops from the urogenital sinus and the surrounding splanchnic mesenchyme. The female urethra and almost all of the male urethra have a similar origin.

Developmental abnormalities of the kidney and excretory passages are relatively common. Early division of the ureteric bud results in bifid or double ureter and supernumerary kidney. Failure of the kidney to ascend from its embryonic position in the pelvis results in ectopic kidney.

The genital or reproductive system develops in close association with the urinary or excretory system. Genetic sex is established at fertilization, but the gonads do not acquire sexual characteristics until the seventh week, and the external genitalia do not become distinctly masculine or feminine until the twelfth week. The genital or reproductive organs in both sexes develop from primordia which appear identical at first. During this *indifferent stage*, an embryo has the potential to develop into a male or female. Gonadal sex is controlled by the Y chromosome which exerts a positive testis-determining action on the *indifferent gonad*. In the presence of a Y chromosome, testes develop and produce masculinizing hormones which stimulate development of the mesonephric ducts into the male genital ducts, and the indifferent external genitalia into the penis and scrotum. These androgens also suppress development of the paramesonephric ducts. In the absence of a Y chromosome and in the presence of two X chromosomes, ovaries develop, the mesonephric ducts regress, the paramesonephric ducts develop into the uterus and uterine tubes, the vagina develops from the urogenital sinus, and the indifferent external genitalia develop into the clitoris and labia.

Errors of the sex-determining mechanism produce true hermaphroditism, an extremely rare condition. Errors in sexual differentiation may cause pseudohermaphroditism. In the male, this results from failure of the fetal testes to produce adequate amounts of masculinizing hormones. In the female, pseudohermaphroditism usually results from a disorder of the fetal adrenal glands which causes an excessive production of androgens.

15

THE CARDIOVASCULAR SYSTEM

The cardiovascular system is the first system to function in the embryo. Blood begins to circulate at the end of the third week. Such early development occurs because the rapidly growing embryo needs an efficient method of acquiring nutrients and disposing of waste products.

DEVELOPMENT OF THE HEART

Heart development is first indicated at 18 or 19 days in the *cardiogenic area* (Fig. 15–

1*A*). A pair of *heart cords* appear and soon become canalized to form endocardial *heart tubes* (Fig. 15–2*B*). The heart tubes approach each other and fuse to form a single median endocardial heart tube (Figs. 15–2*C* and 15–3). With development of the head fold, the heart tube and pericardial cavity come to lie ventral to the foregut and caudal to the oropharyngeal membrane (Fig. 15–4). Concurrently, the heart elongates and develops alternate dilatations and constrictions: the *truncus arteriosus, bulbus cordis, ventricle, atrium* and *sinus venosus* (Fig. 15–3*C*).

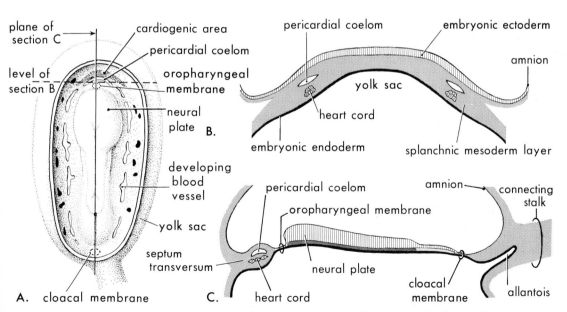

Figure 15–1. *A*, Diagrammatic dorsal view of an embryo of about 19 days showing the cardiogenic area. *B*, Transverse section through the embryo demonstrating the heart cords. *C*, Longitudinal section through the embryo illustrating the relationship of the developing heart to the oropharyngeal (buccopharyngeal) membrane, the pericardial coelom (cavity) and the septum transversum (future central part of the diaphragm).

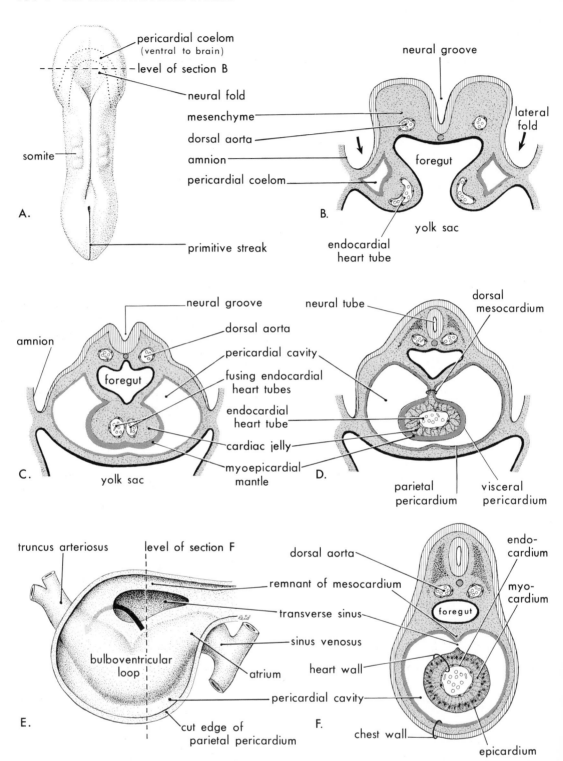

Figure 15–2. *A,* Dorsal view of an embryo of about 20 days. *B,* Transverse section through the heart region showing the widely separated heart tubes and the lateral folds (arrows). *C,* Transverse section through an embryo of about 21 days showing the formation of the pericardial cavity and the heart tubes about to fuse. *D,* Similar section at 22 days showing the single heart tube suspended by the dorsal mesocardium. *E,* Schematic drawing of the heart at about 28 days showing degeneration of the dorsal mesocardium and formation of the transverse pericardial sinus. *F,* Transverse section through this embryo after disappearance of the dorsal mesocardium, showing the layers of the heart wall.

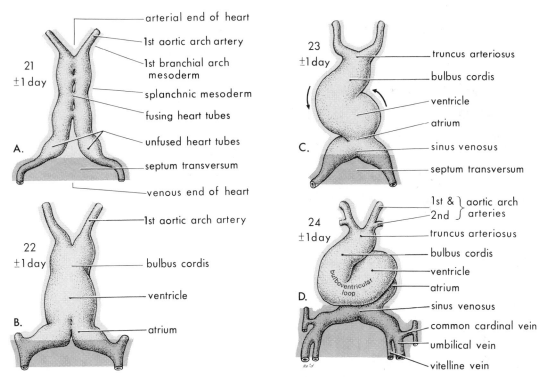

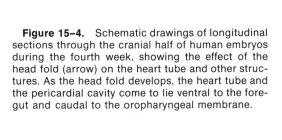

Figure 15–3. Sketches of ventral views of the developing heart during the fourth week, showing fusion of the heart tubes and bending of the single heart tube.

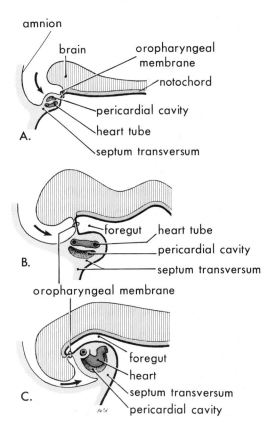

Figure 15–4. Schematic drawings of longitudinal sections through the cranial half of human embryos during the fourth week, showing the effect of the head fold (arrow) on the heart tube and other structures. As the head fold develops, the heart tube and the pericardial cavity come to lie ventral to the foregut and caudal to the oropharyngeal membrane.

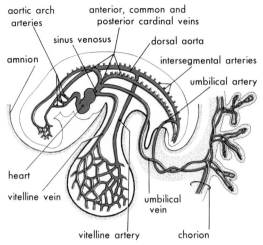

Figure 15–5. Sketch of the cardiovascular system on a 26-day embryo showing vessels of the left side only.

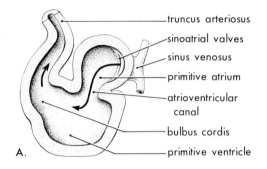

A.

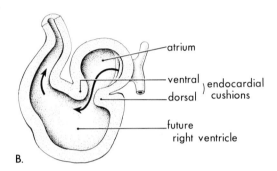

B.

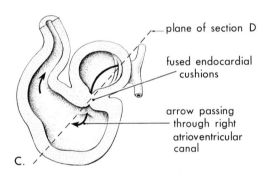

C.

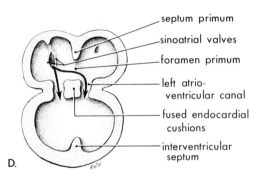

D.

The sinus venosus is a large venous sinus which receives blood from the *umbilical, vitelline* and *common cardinal veins* (Figs. 15–3D and 15–5). Initially the heart is a fairly straight tube, but it soon bends upon itself, forming a U-shaped *bulboventricular loop* (Figs. 15–2E and 15–3D).

DEVELOPMENT OF THE ATRIA AND VENTRICLES

The primitive heart has only one of each chamber. Partitioning of the atrioventricular canal, the atrium and the ventricle begins around the middle of the fourth week and is essentially complete by the end of the fifth week. Although described separately, these processes occur concurrently.

Partitioning of the Atrioventricular Canal. Endocardial cushions develop in the dorsal and ventral walls of the heart in the region of the atrioventricular canal (Fig. 15–6B). These cushions grow toward each other and fuse (Fig. 15–6C), dividing the atrioventricular canal into *right and left atrioventricular canals* (Fig. 15–6D).

Partitioning of the Atrium. A crescent-shaped membrane, the septum primum, grows from the dorsocranial wall of the primitive atrium (Figs. 15–7B and 15–8A). A large opening, the *foramen primum*, exists between its lower free edge and the endocardial cushions. As the septum primum grows toward the endocardial cushions, it

Figure 15–6. *A* to *C*, Sketches of sagittal sections of the heart during the fourth and fifth weeks illustrating division of the atrioventricular canal. *D*, Frontal section of the heart at the plane shown in *C*. The interatrial and interventricular septa have also started to develop.

(Text continued on page 170.)

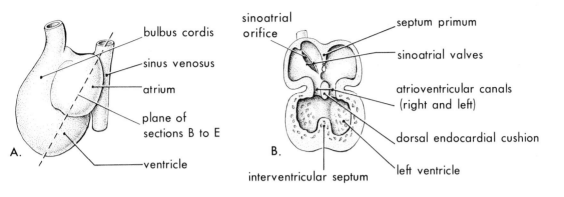

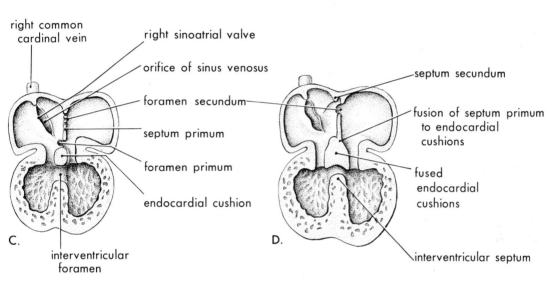

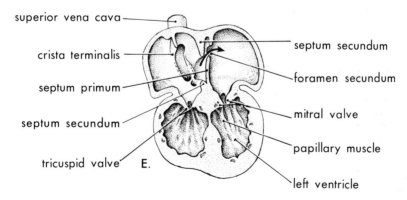

Figure 15–7. Drawings of the developing heart showing partitioning of the atrioventricular canal, the atrium and the ventricle. *A,* Sketch showing the plane of frontal sections *B* to *D. B,* About 28 days, showing the early appearance of the septum primum, the interventricular septum and the dorsal endocardial cushion. *C,* About 30 days, showing perforations in the dorsal part of the septum. *D,* About 35 days, showing the foramen secundum. *E,* About eight weeks, showing the heart after partitioning into four chambers. (Adapted from various sources, especially Patten, 1968.)

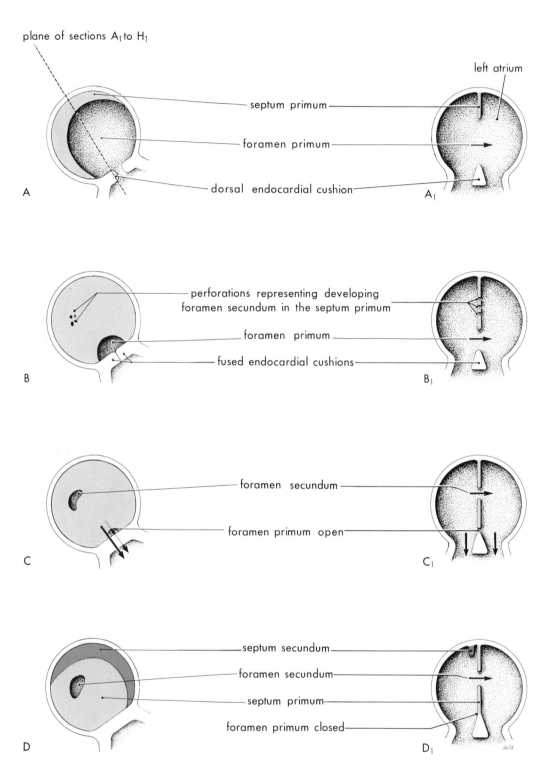

plane of sections A_1 to H_1

septum primum

foramen primum

dorsal endocardial cushion

left atrium

A

A_1

perforations representing developing
foramen secundum in the septum primum

foramen primum

fused endocardial cushions

B

B_1

foramen secundum

foramen primum open

C

C_1

septum secundum

foramen secundum

septum primum

foramen primum closed

D

D_1

Figure 15–8. Diagrammatic sketches illustrating partitioning of the primitive atrium. *A* to *H* are views of the developing interatrial septum as viewed from the right side. A_1 to H_1 are frontal sections of the developing interatrial septum at the plane shown in *A*.

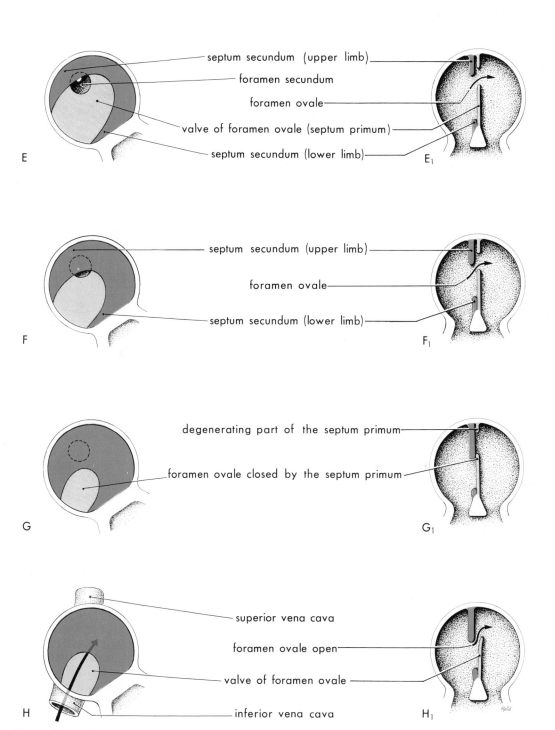

septum secundum (upper limb)

foramen secundum

foramen ovale

valve of foramen ovale (septum primum)

septum secundum (lower limb)

E   E₁

septum secundum (upper limb)

foramen ovale

septum secundum (lower limb)

F   F₁

degenerating part of the septum primum

foramen ovale closed by the septum primum

G   G₁

superior vena cava

foramen ovale open

valve of foramen ovale

inferior vena cava

H   H₁

Figure 15–8. *Continued.*

reduces the size of the foramen primum (Fig. 15–8B and C). Before the foramen primum is obliterated, perforations appear in the upper central part of the septum primum and soon coalesce to form another opening, the *foramen secundum* (Fig. 15–8B to D). Concurrently, the septum primum fuses with the fused endocardial cushions, obliterating the foramen primum.

Subsequently, another crescentic membrane, the *septum secundum,* grows from the ventrocranial wall of the atrium on the right side of the septum primum (Fig. 15–8D). This septum gradually covers the foramen secundum (Fig. 15–8E to G). The oval opening in the septum secundum is called the *foramen ovale* (Fig. 15–8E). The septum primum forms the *valve of the foramen ovale* (Fig. 15–8G_1 and H_1). *Before birth,* the foramen ovale allows most of the blood entering the right atrium to pass into the left atrium (Fig. 15–14). *After birth,* the foramen ovale normally closes and the interatrial septum becomes a complete partition (Fig. 15–15).

Fate of the Sinus Venosus and Formation of the Adult Right Atrium. Initially, the sinus venosus is a separate chamber of the heart and opens into the caudal wall of the right atrium (Figs. 15–5 and 15–6). The *left horn* of the sinus venosus becomes the *coronary sinus* (Fig. 15–9A and B), and the *right horn* of the sinus venosus becomes part of the wall of the *right atrium* (Fig. 15–9B and C).

Formation of the Adult Left Atrium. The smooth part of the wall of the left atrium is derived from the *primitive pulmonary vein.* As the atrium expands, the terminal portion of this vein is gradually absorbed or incorporated into the wall of the left atrium. The remains of the primitive atrium are represented by the auricle.

Partitioning of the Ventricle. Division of the primitive ventricle into right and left ventricles is first indicated by a muscular ridge, the *interventricular septum,* in the floor of the ventricle near its apex (Fig. 15–7B). A crescentic *interventricular foramen* between the free edge of the interventricular septum and the fused endocardial cushions permits communication between the right and left ventricles. The interventricular foramen closes around the end of the seventh week as the result of fusion of tissue from three sources (Fig. 15–11). After closure of the interventricular foramen, the pulmonary trunk is in communication with the right ventricle and the aorta with the left ventricle.

Partitioning of the Truncus Arteriosus. Spirally-arranged ridges form in the truncus arteriosus which fuse to form a spiral *aorticopulmonary septum* (Fig. 15–10D and G). This septum divides the truncus arteriosus into two channels, the *aorta* and the *pulmonary trunk.* The bulbus cordis is gradually incorporated into the walls of the ventricles.

THE AORTIC OR BRANCHIAL ARCH ARTERIES

As the branchial arches develop during the fourth week (see Chapter 11), they receive arteries from the heart. These aortic arch arteries arise from the truncus arteriosus and terminate in the dorsal aorta of the corresponding side (Fig. 15–12B). Although six pairs of aortic arch arteries develop, they are not all present at the same time, e.g., when the sixth pair of aortic arch arteries form, the first two pairs have disappeared (Fig. 15–12C).

Derivatives of the Aortic or Branchial Arch Arteries (Fig. 15–13). During the sixth to eighth weeks, the primitive aortic arch pattern is transformed into the basic adult arterial arrangement. The first and second pairs of aortic arch arteries largely disappear. The proximal parts of the third pair of aortic arch arteries form the *common carotid arteries,* and distal portions join with the dorsal aortae to form the *internal carotid arteries.* The left fourth aortic arch artery forms part of the arch of the aorta. The right fourth aortic arch artery becomes the proximal portion of the *right subclavian artery.* The distal part of this artery forms from the right dorsal aorta and the right seventh intersegmental artery (Fig. 15–13B). The fifth pair of aortic arch arteries have no derivatives. The left sixth aortic arch artery develops as follows: the proximal part persists as the proximal part of the left pulmonary artery, and the distal part persists as a shunt or passageway between the pulmonary artery and the aorta, called the *ductus arteriosus* (Fig. 15–13C and 15–14). The right sixth aortic arch artery develops as follows: the proximal part persists as the proximal part of the right pulmonary artery, and the distal part degenerates.

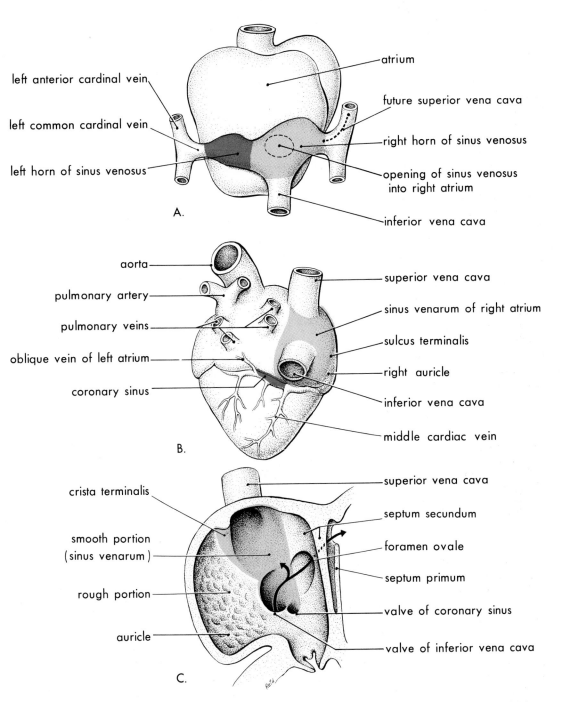

Figure 15–9. Diagrams illustrating the fate of the sinus venosus. *A,* Dorsal view of the heart at about 26 days showing the early appearance of the sinus venosus. *B,* Dorsal view at eight weeks after incorporation of the right horn of the sinus venosus into the right atrium. The left horn of the sinus venosus has become the coronary sinus. *C,* Internal view of the fetal right atrium showing (*1*) the smooth part (sinus venarum) of the wall of the right atrium derived from the right horn of the sinus venosus and (*2*) the crista terminalis and the valves of the interior vena cava and coronary sinus derived from the right sinoatrial valve.

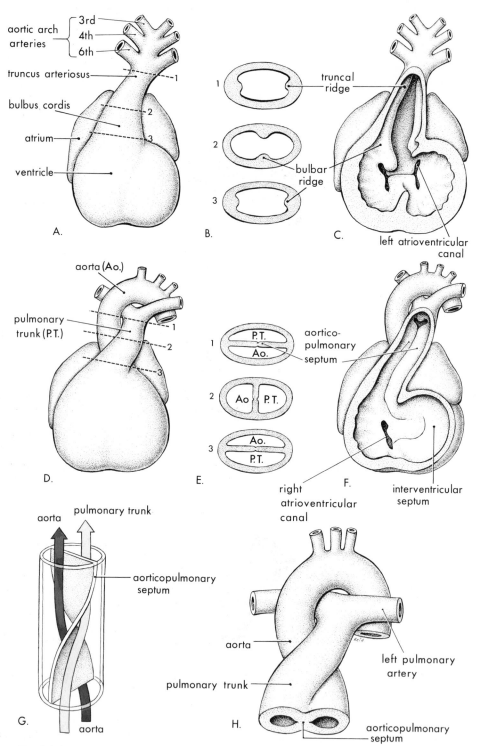

Figure 15–10. Schematic drawings illustrating partitioning of the bulbus cordis and truncus arteriosus. *A,* Ventral aspect of heart at five weeks. *B,* Transverse sections through the truncus arteriosus and bulbus cordis illustrating the truncal and bulbar ridges. *C,* The ventral wall of the heart has been removed to demonstrate the ridges. *D,* Ventral aspect of heart after partitioning of the truncus arteriosus. *E,* Sections through the newly formed aorta (Ao.) and pulmonary trunk (P. T.) showing the aorticopulmonary septum. *F,* Six weeks. The ventral wall of the heart and pulmonary trunk have been removed to show the aorticopulmonary septum. *G,* Diagram illustrating the spiral form of the aorticopulmonary septum. *H,* Drawing showing the great arteries twisting around each other as they leave the heart.

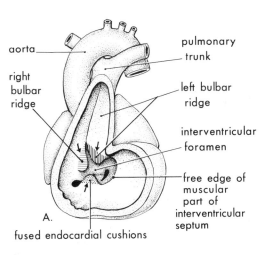

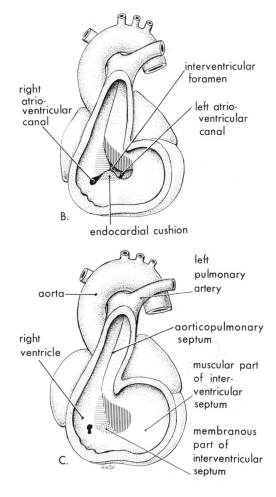

Figure 15-11. Schematic diagrams illustrating closure of the interventricular foramen and formation of the membranous part of the interventricular septum. The walls of the bulbus cordis and the right ventricle have been removed. *A,* 32 days, showing the bulbar ridges and the fused endocardial cushions. *B,* 35 days, showing how proliferation of subendocardial tissue diminishes the interventricular foramen. *C,* Seven weeks, showing the fused bulbar ridges and the membranous part of the interventricular septum formed by extensions of tissue from the right side of the endocardial cushions.

FETAL CIRCULATION

The fetal cardiovascular system is designed to serve prenatal needs and to permit modifications at birth which establish the postnatal circulatory pattern.

Course of the Fetal Circulation (Fig. 15-14). Well-oxygenated blood returns from the placenta in the *umbilical vein.* About half of this blood by-passes the liver, going through the *ductus venosus.* After a short course in the *inferior vena cava,* the blood enters the right atrium. Because the inferior vena cava also contains deoxygenated blood from the lower limbs, abdomen and pelvis, the blood entering the right atrium is not so well oxygenated as that in the umbilical vein. The blood from the inferior vena cava is largely directed by the lower border of the septum secundum through the foramen ovale into the left atrium. Here it mixes with a relatively small amount of deoxygenated blood returning from the lungs via the pulmonary veins. The blood passes into the left ventricle and leaves via the ascending aorta. Consequently, the vessels to the heart, head and neck and upper limbs receive rather well-oxygenated blood.

A small amount of oxygenated blood from the inferior vena cava remains in the right atrium. This blood mixes with deoxygenated blood from the superior vena cava and coronary sinus and passes into the right ventricle. The blood leaves by the pulmonary trunk, most of it passing through the ductus arteriosus into the aorta. Very little blood goes to the lungs because they are nonfunctional and so require little blood. Most of the mixed blood in the descending aorta passes into the umbilical arteries and is returned to the placenta for reoxygenation; the remainder circulates through the lower part of the body and eventually enters the inferior vena cava.

(Text continued on page 178.)

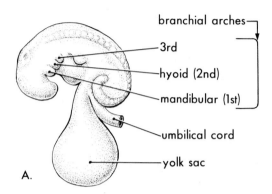

A.

branchial arches
3rd
hyoid (2nd)
mandibular (1st)
umbilical cord
yolk sac

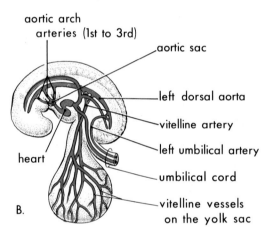

B.

aortic arch
arteries (1st to 3rd)
aortic sac
left dorsal aorta
vitelline artery
left umbilical artery
umbilical cord
vitelline vessels
on the yolk sac
heart

Figure 15–12. Drawings illustrating the aortic arch arteries and the primitive cardiovascular system. *A,* Left side of a 26-day embryo. *B,* Schematic drawing of this embryo showing the left aortic arch arteries arising from the aortic sac of the truncus arteriosus, running through the branchial arches and terminating in the left dorsal aorta. *C,* 35-day embryo showing the single dorsal aorta and that the first two pairs of aortic arch arteries have largely degenerated.

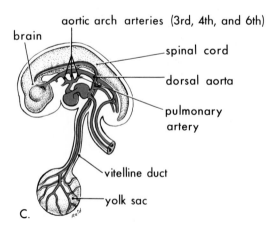

C.

aortic arch arteries (3rd, 4th, and 6th)
brain
spinal cord
dorsal aorta
pulmonary artery
vitelline duct
yolk sac

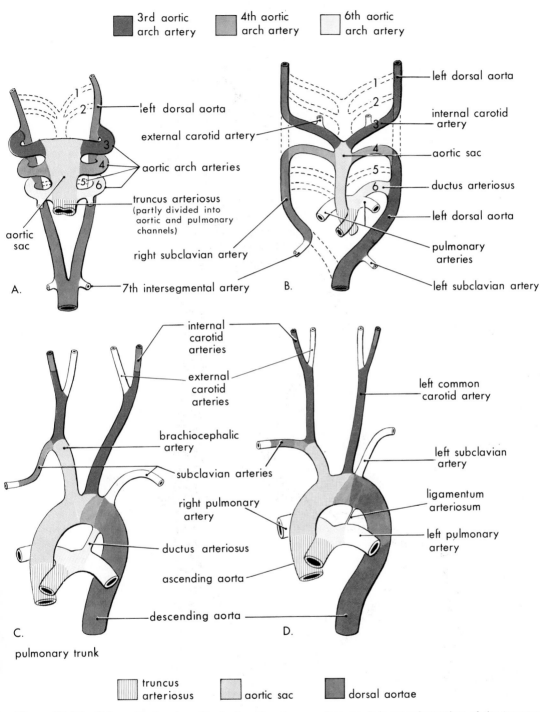

3rd aortic arch artery

4th aortic arch artery

6th aortic arch artery

A.

left dorsal aorta

external carotid artery

aortic arch arteries

truncus arteriosus (partly divided into aortic and pulmonary channels)

aortic sac

right subclavian artery

7th intersegmental artery

B.

left dorsal aorta

internal carotid artery

aortic sac

ductus arteriosus

left dorsal aorta

pulmonary arteries

left subclavian artery

C.

internal carotid arteries

external carotid arteries

brachiocephalic artery

subclavian arteries

right pulmonary artery

ductus arteriosus

ascending aorta

descending aorta

pulmonary trunk

D.

left common carotid artery

left subclavian artery

ligamentum arteriosum

left pulmonary artery

truncus arteriosus

aortic sac

dorsal aortae

Figure 15–13. Schematic drawings illustrating the changes that result in transformation of the truncus arteriosus, aortic sac, aortic arch arteries and dorsal aortae into the adult arterial pattern. The vessels which are not shaded or colored are not derived from these structures. *A,* Aortic arch arteries at six weeks; by this stage the first two pairs of aortic arch arteries have largely disappeared. *B,* Aortic arch arteries at seven weeks; the parts of the dorsal aortae and aortic arches that normally disappear are indicated with broken lines. *C,* Arterial arrangement at eight weeks. *D,* Sketch of the arterial vessels of a six-month infant.

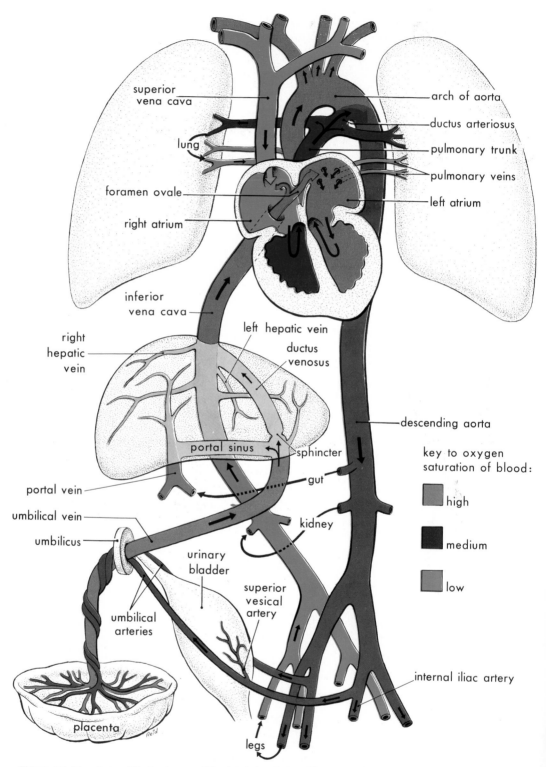

Figure 15–14. A simplified scheme of the fetal circulation. The colors indicate the oxygen saturation of the blood and the arrows show the course of the fetal circulation. The organs are not drawn to scale.

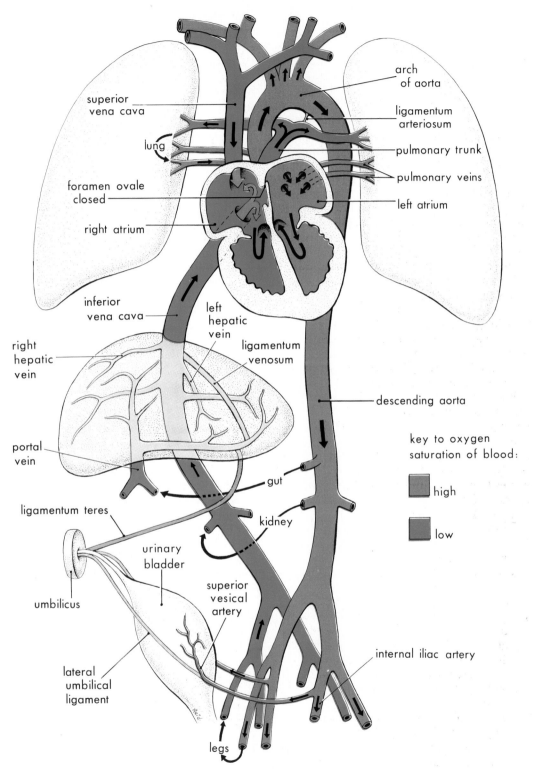

Figure 15–15. A simplified representation of the circulation after birth. The adult derivatives of the fetal vessels and structures that become nonfunctional at birth are also shown. The arrows indicate the course of the neonatal circulation. The organs are not drawn to scale.

Changes in the Cardiovascular System at Birth (Fig. 15–15). Important circulatory adjustments occur at birth when the circulation of fetal blood through the placenta ceases and the lungs begin to function. The foramen ovale, the ductus arteriosus, the ductus venosus and the umbilical vessels are no longer needed. Occlusion of the placental circulation causes an immediate fall of blood pressure in the inferior vena cava and the right atrium. Aeration of the lungs is associated with a dramatic fall in pulmonary vascular resistance, a marked increase in pulmonary blood flow, and a progressive thinning of the walls of the pulmonary arteries. As a result of this increased pulmonary blood flow, the pressure in the left atrium is raised above that in the right atrium. This closes the foramen ovale by pressing its valve, the septum primum, against the septum secundum (Fig. 15–15).

The ductus arteriosus and the umbilical arteries constrict at birth. The closure of the fetal vessels and the foramen ovale is initially a functional change; later there is anatomical closure resulting from proliferation of endothelial and fibrous tissues.

Because of the changes in the cardiovascular system at birth, certain vessels and structures are no longer required. They are transformed as follows (Fig. 15–15):

The intra-abdominal portion of the umbilical vein forms the *ligamentum teres,* which passes from the umbilicus to the left branch of the portal vein.

The ductus venosus becomes the *ligamentum venosum,* which passes through the liver from the left branch of the portal vein to the inferior vena cava.

Most of the intra-abdominal portions of the umbilical arteries form the *lateral umbilical ligaments;* the proximal parts of these vessels persist as the *superior vesical arteries.*

The foramen ovale normally closes functionally at birth. Later anatomical closure results from tissue proliferation and adhesion of the septum primum (the valve of the foramen ovale) to the left margin of the septum secundum.

The ductus arteriosus becomes the *ligamentum arteriosum,* which passes from the left pulmonary artery to the arch of the aorta. Anatomical closure of the ductus normally occurs by the end of the third postnatal month.

CONGENITAL MALFORMATIONS OF THE HEART AND GREAT VESSELS

Because development of the heart and great vessels is complex, congenital heart defects are relatively common. The overall incidence is about 0.7 per cent of live births and 2.7 per cent of stillbirths.

The following malformations are relatively common and many are amenable to surgery:

Atrial Septal Defects (ASD) (Fig. 15–16). Atrial septal defect is among the most common of congenital heart defects. There are two main types:

Secundum type ASD (Fig. 15–16A to D). The defect is in the area of the foramen ovale and may include defects of the septum primum and of the septum secundum. Patent foramen ovale may result from abnormal resorption of the septum primum during the formation of the foramen secundum. If resorption occurs in abnormal locations, the septum primum is fenestrated or net-like (Fig. 15–16A). If excessive resorption of the septum primum occurs, the resulting short septum primum does not cover the foramen ovale (Fig. 15–16B). If an abnormally large foramen ovale results from defective development of the septum secundum, a normal septum primum will not close the foramen ovale at birth (Fig. 15–16C). Large atrial septal defects may result from a combination of excessive resorption of the septum primum and a large foramen ovale (Fig. 15–16D).

Endocardial cushion defect with primum type ASD (Fig. 15–16E). The septum primum does not fuse with the endocardial cushions, leaving a *patent foramen primum;* usually there is also a cleft in the mitral valve.

Ventricular Septal Defects (VSD). This relatively common abnormality ranks first in frequency on all lists of cardiac defects. Membranous septal defect is the commonest type of VSD (Fig. 15–17B). Incomplete closure of the interventricular foramen and failure of the membranous septum to develop result from failure of extensions of subendocardial tissue to grow from the right side of the fused endocardial cushions and fuse with the aorticopulmonary septum and the muscular part of the interventricu-

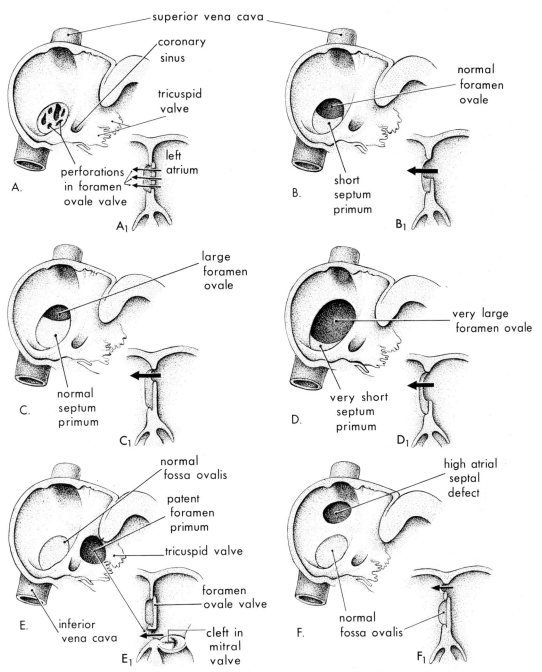

Figure 15–16. Drawings of the right aspect of the interatrial septum (*A* to *F*) and sketches of frontal sections through the septum (*A₁* to *F₁*) illustrating various types of atrial septal defect. *A,* Patent foramen ovale resulting from resorption of the septum primum in abnormal locations. *B,* Patent foramen ovale caused by excessive resorption of the septum primum, sometimes called the "short flap defect." *C,* Patent foramen ovale resulting from an abnormally large foramen ovale. *D,* Patent foramen ovale resulting from (1) an abnormally large foramen ovale, and (2) excessive resorption of the septum primum. *E,* Endocardial cushion defect with primum type atrial septal defect. The frontal section E₁ also shows the cleft in the septal leaflet of the mitral valve. *F,* High septal defect resulting from abnormal absorption of the sinus venosus into the right atrium. This is a very rare defect. Note the fossa ovalis in *E* and *F* which forms when the foramen ovale closes normally.

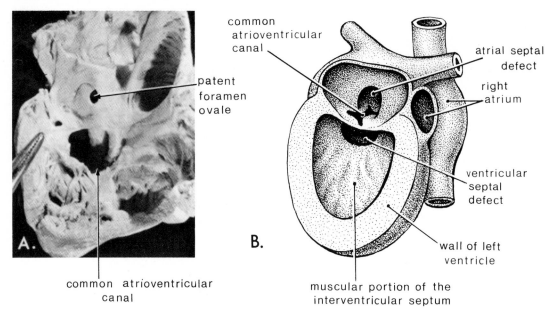

Figure 15–17. *A,* Photograph of an infant's heart, sectioned and viewed from the right side, showing a patent foramen ovale and a common atrioventricular canal. (From Lev, M.: *Autopsy Diagnosis of Congenitally Malformed Hearts.* 1953. Courtesy of Charles C Thomas, Publisher, Springfield, Illinois.) *B,* Schematic drawing of a heart illustrating various defects of the cardiac septa.

lar septum (Fig. 15–11*C*). VSD is often associated with other defects of the cardiac septa (Fig. 15–17).

Persistent Truncus Arteriosus. This malformation results from failure of development of the aorticopulmonary septum. As a result the truncus arteriosus does not divide into the aorta and pulmonary trunk. The most common type is a single arterial vessel which gives rise to the pulmonary trunk and ascending aorta (Fig. 15–18*A* and *B*). The next most common type is for the right and left pulmonary arteries to arise close together from the dorsal wall of the persistent truncus arteriosus (Fig. 15–18*C*). Less common types of persistent truncus arteriosus are illustrated in Figure 15–18*D* and *E*.

Complete Transposition of the Great Arteries (Vessels). In typical cases, the aorta lies anterior to the pulmonary trunk and arises from the right ventricle; the pulmonary trunk arises from the left ventricle. For survival, there must be an associated septal defect or patent ductus arteriosus to permit some interchange of blood between the pulmonary and systemic circulations. During partitioning of the truncus arteriosus, the aorticopulmonary septum fails to pursue a

spiral course. As a result the origins of the great arteries are reversed.

Tetralogy of Fallot (Fig. 15–19*B*). This is a combination of four cardiac defects consisting of (1) pulmonary stenosis or narrowing of the region of the right ventricular outflow (pulmonary valve), (2) ventricular septal defect, (3) overriding aorta and (4) hypertrophy of the right ventricle. This condition results in cyanosis or blueness of the lips and fingernails; these infants are sometimes referred to as "blue babies."

Aortic Arch Anomalies

Because of the many changes involved in transformation of the embryonic aortic arch system into the adult arterial pattern, it is understandable that variations may occur. Abnormalities result from the persistence of parts of aortic arch arteries which normally disappear, from disappearance of other parts which normally persist or from both.

Coarctation of the Aorta (Fig. 15–20). This relatively common malformation is characterized by a narrowing of the aorta, usually just above or below the ductus ar-

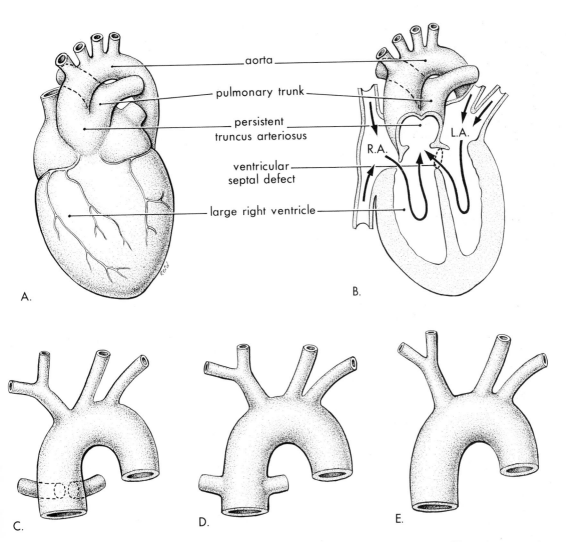

aorta

pulmonary trunk

persistent
truncus arteriosus

ventricular
septal defect

large right ventricle

R.A.

L.A.

A.

B.

C.

D.

E.

Figure 15–18. Drawings illustrating the main types of persistent truncus arteriosus. *A,* The common trunk divides into an aorta and short pulmonary trunk. *B,* Sketch showing circulation in this heart and a ventricular septal defect. *C,* The right and left pulmonary arteries arise close together from the truncus arteriosus. *D,* The pulmonary arteries arise independently from the sides of the truncus arteriosus. *E,* No pulmonary arteries are present; in such cases the lungs are supplied by bronchial arteries.

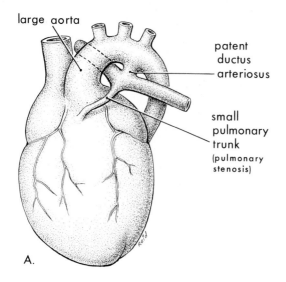

large aorta

patent
ductus
arteriosus

small
pulmonary
trunk
(pulmonary
stenosis)

A.

Figure 15-19. *A,* Drawing of an infant's heart showing a small pulmonary trunk (pulmonary stenosis) and a large aorta resulting from unequal partitioning of the truncus arteriosus. There is also hypertrophy of the right ventricle and a patent ductus arteriosus. *B,* Frontal section of a heart illustrating the tetralogy of Fallot. Note that the large aorta lies over the VSD and receives blood from both ventricles.

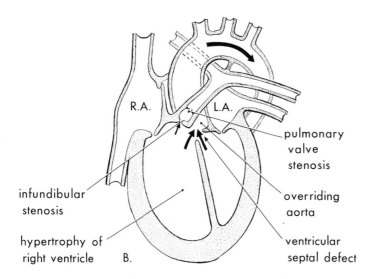

R.A.   L.A.

pulmonary
valve
stenosis

infundibular
stenosis

overriding
aorta

hypertrophy of
right ventricle   B.

ventricular
septal defect

teriosus. The embryological basis of coarctation of the aorta is unclear. There is an abnormal involution of a small segment of the left dorsal aorta (Fig. 15–20*F*). Later this stenotic segment (area of coarctation) moves cranially with the left subclavian artery to the region of the ductus arteriosus (Fig. 15–20*G*).

Postductal coarctation. In this common type, the constriction is below the level of the ductus arteriosus (Fig. 15–20*A*). A collateral circulation develops during the fetal period, thus assisting with passage of blood to lower parts of the body (Fig. 15–20*B*).

Preductal coarctation. In this less common type, the constriction is above the level

of the ductus arteriosus (Fig. 15–20*C*). The ductus usually remains open, providing a communication between the pulmonary artery and the descending aorta. The narrowed segment is occasionally long (Fig. 15–20*D*).

Patent Ductus Arteriosus (Fig. 15–21). This malformation is two to three times more common in females than in males. The embryological basis of patent ductus arteriosus is failure of the ductus arteriosus, joining the pulmonary artery and the aorta, to involute after birth and form the ligamentum arteriosum. Patent ductus arteriosus is the commonest cardiac malformation associated with maternal rubella infection during early pregnancy (see Chapter 9).

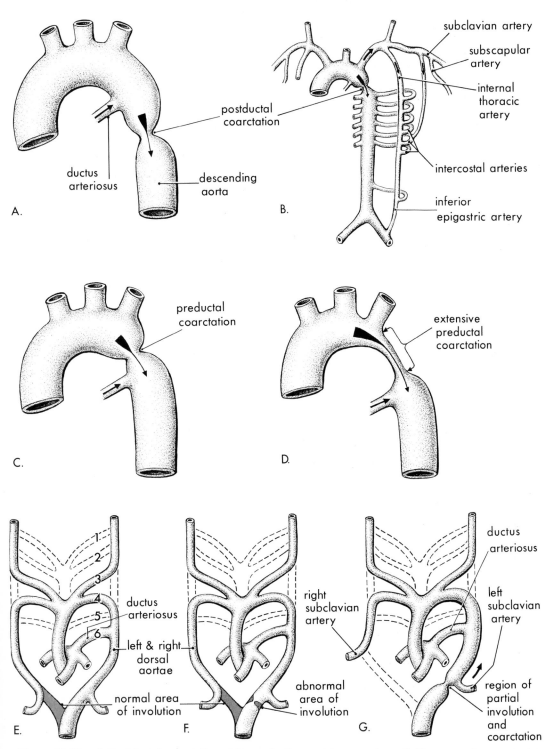

Figure 15–20. *A,* Postductal coarctation of the aorta, the most common type. *B,* Diagrammatic representation of the common routes of collateral circulation that develop in association with coarctation of the aorta. *C* and *D,* Preductal coarctation. The type illustrated in *D* is usually associated with major cardiac defects. *E,* Sketch of the aortic arch pattern in a seven-week embryo showing the areas that normally involute. Note that the distal segment of the right dorsal aorta normally involutes as the right subclavian artery develops. *F,* Localized abnormal involution of a small distal segment of the left dorsal aorta. *G,* Later stage showing the abnormally involuted segment appearing as a coarctation of the aorta. This moves (arrow) to the region of the ductus arteriosus with the left subclavian artery.

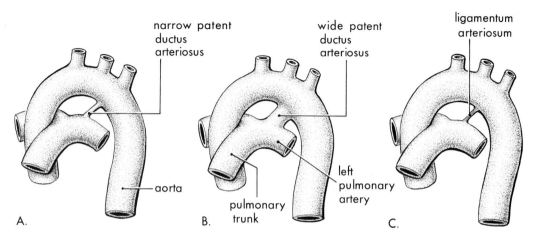

Figure 15–21. *A,* The ductus arteriosus of a newborn infant. The ductus is normally patent for about two weeks after birth. *B,* Abnormal patent ductus arteriosus in a six-month infant. In this case, some of the blood that should go through the aorta to the lower part of the body goes back to the lungs via the ductus arteriosus and the pulmonary arteries. The ductus is nearly the same size as the left pulmonary artery. *C,* The ligamentum arteriosum, normal remnant of the ductus arteriosus, in a six-month infant.

SUMMARY

The cardiovascular system begins to develop during the third week from splanchnic mesoderm. Paired heart tubes form and fuse into a single heart tube. By the end of the third week, a functional cardiovascular system is present. As the heart tube grows, it bends to the right and soon acquires the general external appearance of the adult heart. The heart becomes partitioned into four chambers during the fourth and fifth weeks. The critical period of heart development is from about day 20 to day 50. Because partitioning of the heart is complex, *defects of the cardiac septa are relatively common,* particularly ventricular septal defects. Some congenital malformations result from abnormal transformation of the aortic (branchial) arch arteries into the adult arterial pattern.

Because the lungs are nonfunctional during prenatal life, the fetal cardiovascular system is structurally designed so that blood is oxygenated at the placenta and largely bypasses the lungs. The modifications which establish the postnatal circulatory pattern at birth are not abrupt, but extend into infancy. Failure of the normal changes in the circulatory system to occur at birth results in a *patent foramen ovale* or a *patent ductus arteriosus* or both.

16

THE SKELETAL AND MUSCULAR SYSTEMS

THE SKELETAL SYSTEM

The skeletal system develops from mesoderm, the formation of which is described in Chapter 5. Most bones first appear as mesenchymal condensations and then as hyaline cartilage models which become ossified by endochondral ossification. Some bones develop in mesenchyme by intramembranous bone formation.[1]

The Axial Skeleton

Vertebral Column and Ribs
Precartilaginous stage. During the fourth week, mesenchymal cells from the somites migrate in three main directions (Fig. 16–1D):

1. Cells move ventromedially to surround the notochord. The body of each vertebra develops from the caudal part of one somite together with the cranial portion of the next somite. The notochord eventually degenerates and disappears where it is surrounded by the developing vertebral body. Between the vertebrae it expands to form the gelatinous center of the intervertebral disc, called the *nucleus pulposus.*

---

[1] For details of bone formation, see a histology textbook.

2. Cells migrate dorsally to cover the neural tube. These mesenchymal cells give rise to the *vertebral* or *neural arch* of the vertebra.

3. Cells pass ventrolaterally into the body wall and form the costal processes which develop into ribs in the thoracic region.

THE SKULL

The skull develops from mesenchyme around the developing brain. It consists of the *neurocranium*, a protective case for the brain, and the *viscerocranium*, the main skeleton of the jaws.

The Neurocranium

Cartilaginous Neurocranium (Chondrocranium). Initially, this consists of the cartilaginous base of the developing skull which forms by fusion of several cartilages (Fig. 16–2). Later, endochondral ossification of this chondrocranium forms various bones in the base of the skull.

Membranous Neurocranium. Intramembranous ossification occurs in the mesenchyme investing the brain and forms the bones of the cranial vault (Fig. 16–2D). During fetal life and infancy, the flat bones of

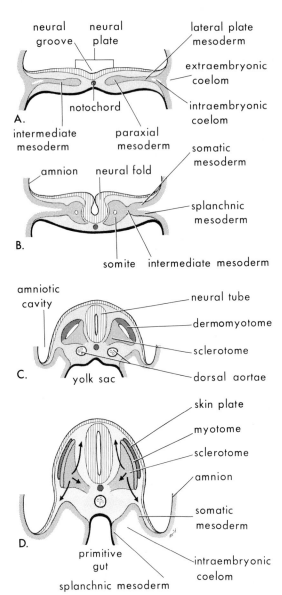

Figure 16-1. Transverse sections through embryos of various ages illustrating the formation and early differentiation of somites. See Figure 6-4 for the external appearance of these embryos. *A*, Presomite embryo showing the paraxial mesoderm from which the somites are derived. *B*, Embryo of about 22 days. *C*, Embryo of about 26 days. The dermomyotome region of the somite gives rise to a myotome. *D*, Embryo of about 28 days. The arrows indicate the migration of cells from the sclerotome regions of the somites.

the skull are separated by dense connective tissue membranes or fibrous joints called *sutures* (Fig. 16-3). Six large fibrous areas, the "soft spots" called *fontanelles*, are also

present. The softness of the bones and their loose connections at the sutures enable the skull to undergo changes of shape during birth, called *molding* (e.g., the forehead becomes flattened and the occiput (back of the head) drawn out as the bones overlap). This construction also enables the skull to enlarge rapidly with the brain during infancy and childhood.

The Viscerocranium

Cartilaginous Viscerocranium (Fig. 16-2*D*). This consists of the cartilaginous skeleton of the first three *branchial arches* (see Chapter 11). During endochondral ossification, the dorsal end of the *first arch cartilage* (Meckel's cartilage) forms two middle ear bones, the malleus and incus (Fig. 16-2*D*). The dorsal end of the *second arch cartilage* (Reichert's cartilage) forms the stapes of the middle ear and the styloid process of the temporal bone. The ventral end ossifies to form the lesser cornu and upper part of the body of the hyoid bone. The ventral end of the *third arch cartilage* gives rise to the greater cornu and lower part of the body of the hyoid bone (Fig. 16-2*D*).

Membranous Viscerocranium (Fig. 16-2*D*). Intramembranous ossification occurs within the maxillary process of the first branchial or mandibular arch and forms the premaxilla, the maxilla, the zygomatic and the squamous temporal bones. The mesenchyme of the mandibular process of this arch condenses around the first arch cartilage (Meckel's cartilage) and undergoes intramembranous ossification to form the mandible. This cartilage disappears ventral to the portion which forms the sphenomandibular ligament. Thus Meckel's cartilage does not give rise to the adult mandible.

The Newborn Skull. The skull at birth is like the fetal skull (Fig. 16-3); it is rather round and its bones are quite thin. The skull is large in proportion to the rest of the skeleton, and the face is relatively small compared with the cranium. The small facial region results from the small size of the jaws, the virtual absence of paranasal air sinuses and the general underdevelopment of the facial bones.

Postnatal Growth of the Skull. Growth of the cranial vault, especially during the first year, is rapid and continues until the sev-

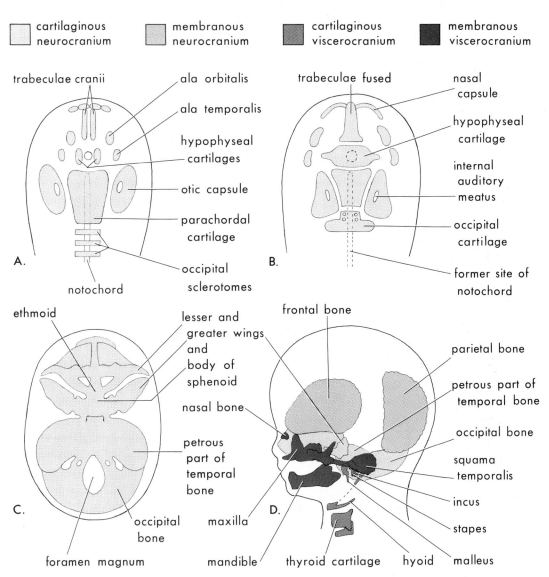

cartilaginous
neurocranium

membranous
neurocranium

cartilaginous
viscerocranium

membranous
viscerocranium

trabeculae cranii

ala orbitalis

ala temporalis

hypophyseal
cartilages

otic capsule

parachordal
cartilage

A.

occipital
sclerotomes

notochord

trabeculae fused

nasal
capsule

hypophyseal
cartilage

internal
auditory
meatus

occipital
cartilage

B.

former site of
notochord

ethmoid

lesser and
greater wings
and
body of
sphenoid

frontal bone

parietal bone

petrous part of
temporal bone

occipital bone

squama
temporalis

incus

stapes

malleus

nasal bone

petrous
part of
temporal
bone

C.

occipital
bone

foramen magnum

maxilla

mandible

D.

thyroid cartilage

hyoid

Figure 16–2. Diagrams illustrating stages in the development of the skull. *A* to *C* are viewed from above; *D* is a lateral view. *A,* Six weeks, showing the various cartilages that will fuse to form the chondrocranium. *B,* Seven weeks, after fusion of some of the paired cartilages. *C,* 12 weeks, showing the cartilaginous base of the skull or chondrocranium formed by the fusion of various cartilages. *D,* 20 weeks, indicating the derivation of the bones of the fetal skull.

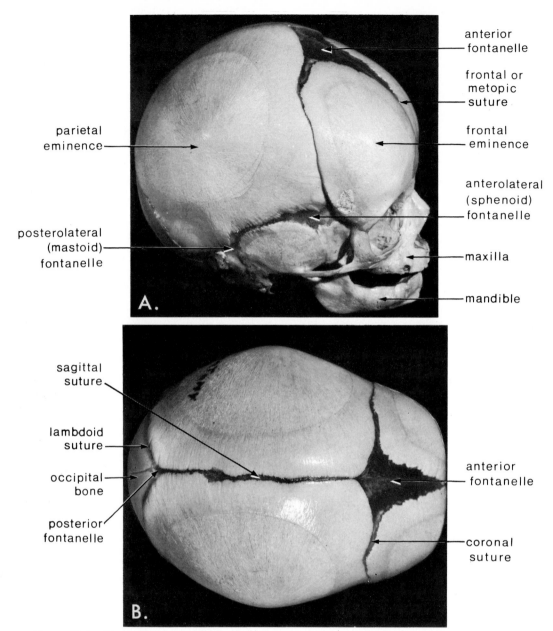

Figure 16-3. Photographs of a fetal skull showing the fontanelles, the bones and the connecting sutures. *A,* Lateral view. *B,* Superior view. The posterior and anterolateral fontanelles close within two to three months after birth by growth of the surrounding bones. The posterolateral fontanelles close similarly by the end of the first year, and the anterior fontanelle closes about the middle of the second year. The two halves of the frontal bone normally begin to fuse during the second year, and the frontal or metopic suture is often obliterated by the eighth year. The other sutures begin to disappear during adult life, but the times when the sutures close are subject to wide variations.

enth year. This growth is related to the rapid development of the brain. There is also rapid growth of the face and jaws, coinciding with the eruption of the primary or deciduous teeth; these changes are still more marked after the permanent teeth erupt (see Chapter 19). There is concurrent enlargement of the frontal and facial regions associated with the increase in the size of the paranasal air sinuses.

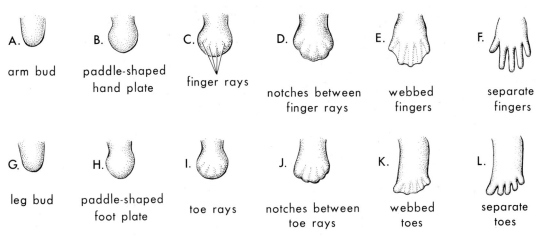

Figure 16–4. Drawings illustrating stages in the development of the hands and feet between the fourth and eighth weeks.

THE APPENDICULAR SKELETON

The appendicular skeleton consists of the pectoral (shoulder) and pelvic girdles and the limb bones. The general features of early limb development are described and illustrated in Chapter 6. The *limb buds* first appear as small elevations of the ventrolateral body wall toward the end of the fourth week. The early stages of limb development are alike for the upper and lower limbs (Figs. 16–4 and 16–5), except that development of the *arm buds* precedes that of the *leg buds* by a few days. The arm buds develop opposite the caudal cervical segments, and the leg buds form opposite the lumbar and upper sacral segments. Each limb bud consists of a mass of mesenchyme derived from the somatic mesoderm and is covered by a layer of ectoderm. The *apical ectodermal ridge* (Fig. 16–6B) exerts an inductive influence on this mesenchyme which promotes growth and development of the limbs. The ends of the flipper-like limb buds flatten into paddle-like hand or foot plates, and digits differentiate at the margins of these plates (Fig. 16–4).

As the limbs elongate and the bones form, myoblasts (muscle-forming cells) aggregate and develop into a large muscle mass in each extremity. In general, this muscle mass separates into dorsal (extensor) and ventral (flexor) components. Initially, the limbs are directed caudally; later they extend ventrally, and then the developing arms and legs rotate in opposite directions and to different degrees (Fig. 16–5). Originally, the flexor aspect of the limbs is ventral and the

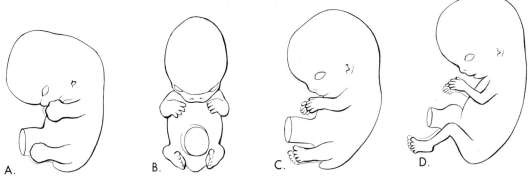

Figure 16–5. Drawings illustrating positional changes of the developing limbs: *A*, About 37 days, showing the extremities extending ventrally and the hand and foot plates facing each other. *B*, About 41 days, showing the arms bent at the elbows and the hands curved over the thorax. *C*, About 43 days, showing the soles of the feet facing each other. *D*, About 48 days. Note that the elbows now point caudally and the knees cranially.

☐ loose mesenchyme   ▦ condensed mesenchyme   ■ cartilage

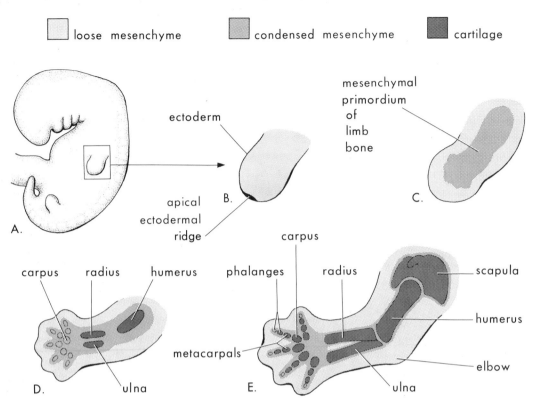

Figure 16–6. *A,* An embryo of about 28 days, showing the early appearance of the limb buds. *B,* Schematic drawing of a longitudinal section through an early arm bud. The apical ectodermal ridge has an inductive influence on the loose mesenchyme in the limb bud; it promotes growth of the mesenchyme and appears to give it the ability to form specific cartilaginous elements. *C,* Similar sketch of an arm bud at 33 days showing the mesenchymal primordium of a limb bone. *D,* Forelimb at six weeks showing the hyaline cartilage models of the various bones. *E,* Later in the sixth week, showing the completed cartilaginous models of the bones of the upper limb.

extensor aspect dorsal. The arm buds rotate laterally through 90° on their longitudinal axes; thus the future elbows point backward or dorsally, and the extensor muscles come to lie on the outer and dorsal aspect of the arm. The leg buds rotate medially through almost 90°; thus the future knees point forward or ventrolaterally, and the extensor muscles lie on the ventral aspect of the leg. It should also be clear that the radius and tibia and the ulna and fibula are homologous bones, just as the thumb and the big toe are homologous digits.

During the sixth week, the mesenchymal primordia of bones in the limb buds undergo chondrification to form hyaline cartilage models of the future appendicular skeleton (Fig. 16–6*D* and *E*). The models of the pectoral girdle and the upper limb bones appear slightly before those of the pelvic girdle and lower limbs, and the models of each extremity appear in a proximodistal sequence. Ossification begins in the long bones by the end of the embryonic period; by 12 weeks primary centers have appeared in nearly all bones of the extremities. Secondary centers of ossification appear after birth.

THE MUSCULAR SYSTEM

The muscular system also develops from mesoderm. Muscle tissue develops from primitive cells called *myoblasts.*

Skeletal Musculature

The myoblasts which form the skeletal musculature are derived from the myotome regions of the somites, the branchial arches and the somatic mesoderm. The myoblasts elongate, aggregate to form parallel bundles and then fuse to form multinucleated cells. During early fetal life, myofibrils appear in the cytoplasm and show the characteristic cross striations by the end of the third month.

The migration of myoblasts from the branchial arches to form the muscles of mastication, of facial expression and of the pharynx and larynx is described in Chapter 11. Myoblasts from the *occipital myotomes* form the tongue muscles.

The musculature of the limbs develops from the mesenchyme surrounding the developing bones. It is now generally believed that there is no migration of mesenchyme from the somites to form limb muscles.

Visceral Musculature

Smooth Muscle. Smooth muscle differentiates from splanchnic mesoderm surrounding the primitive gut and its derivatives (see Chapter 13). Elsewhere, smooth muscle develops from mesenchyme in the area concerned. The myoblasts elongate and develop contractile elements. The muscles of the iris and the myoepithelial cells of mammary and sweat glands appear to be derived from mesenchymal cells that originate from the ectoderm.

Cardiac Muscle. Cardiac muscle develops from splanchnic mesoderm surrounding the heart (see Chapter 15). The myoblasts adhere to each other, as in developing skeletal muscle, but the intervening cell membranes do not disintegrate. These areas of adhesion become the *intercalated discs.* Usually there is a single central nucleus, and myofibrils develop as in skeletal muscle cells. Late in the embryonic period, special bundles of muscle cells develop with relatively few myofibrils and relatively larger diameters than typical cardiac muscle cells. These atypical cardiac muscle cells, called *Purkinje fibers*, later form the conducting system of the heart.

CONGENITAL MALFORMATIONS OF THE SKELETAL AND MUSCULAR SYSTEMS

Acrania. In this condition, the cranial vault is absent and a large spinal defect is usually present (Fig. 16–7). Acrania is as-

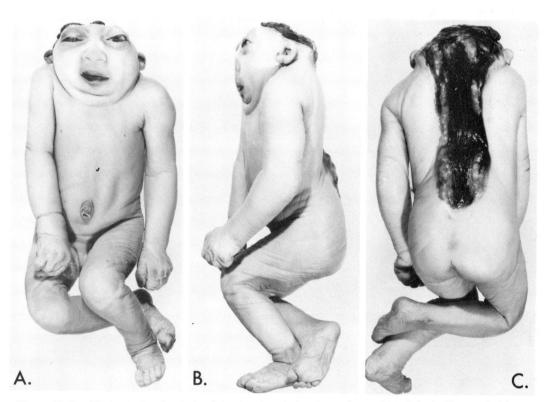

Figure 16–7. Photographs of anterior, lateral and posterior views of a newborn infant with acrania (absence of cranial vault), anencephaly (absence of forebrain), rachischisis (extensive cleft in vertebral column) and myeloschisis (severe malformation of the spinal cord).

sociated with anencephaly (absence of most of the brain); this condition is discussed in Chapter 17.

Spina Bifida Occulta. This defect of the vertebral column results from failure of fusion of the halves of the vertebral arch. It is commonly observed in roentgenograms of the lumbar or sacral region. Frequently, only one vertebra is affected. Although this is a common vertebral defect, it is usually of no significance. The skin over the bifid spine is intact and there may be no external evidence of the defect; sometimes the malformation is indicated by a dimple or a tuft of hair (see Figure 17–19). Severe types of spina bifida are discussed in Chapter 17 with congenital malformations of the nervous system.

Malformations of the Limbs

Minor defects are relatively common, but major limb malformations are generally rare. An "epidemic" of limb deformities occurred from 1957 to 1962 as a result of maternal ingestion of thalidomide (Fig. 16–8). This drug was withdrawn in 1961.

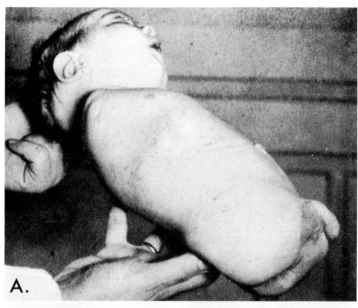

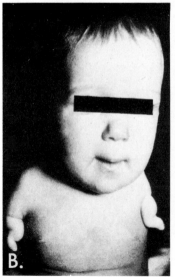

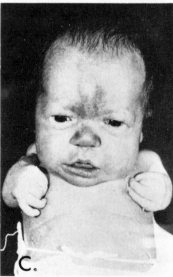

Figure 16–8. Limb malformations caused by thalidomide. *A,* Quadruple amelia. The upper and lower limbs are absent. *B,* meromelia of the upper limbs. The arms are represented by rudimentary stumps. *C,* Meromelia, with the rudimentary upper limbs attached directly to the trunk. (From Lenz, W., and Knapp, K.: *German Med. Monthly* 7:253, 1962.)

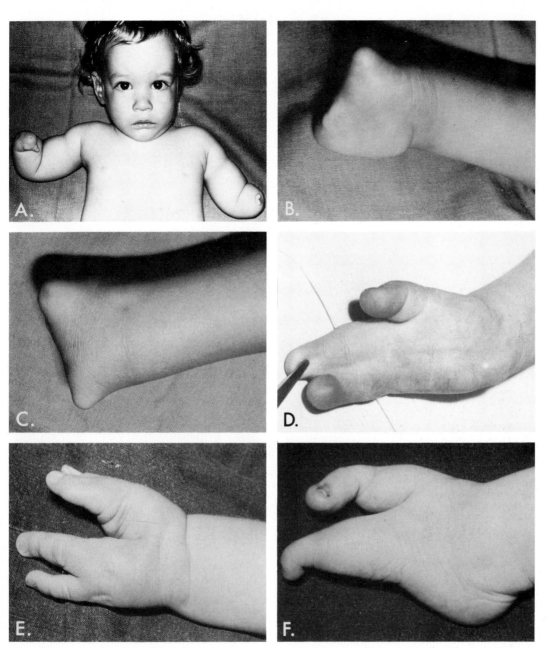

Figure 16-9. Photographs illustrating various types of meromelia. *A,* Absence of the hands and most of the forearms. *B,* Absence of the phalanges. *C,* Absence of the hand. *D,* Absence of the fourth and fifth phalanges and metacarpals. There is also syndactyly. *E,* Absence of the third phalanx, resulting in a cleft hand (lobster claw). *F,* Absence of the second and third toes, resulting in a cleft foot. (*D* is from Swenson, O.: *Pediatric Surgery,* 1958. Courtesy of Appleton-Century-Crofts, Inc.)

Absence of the Hands and Phalanges (Fig. 16-9*A* to *D*). Absence of the fingers, and often part of the hand, is not too common. Often genetic factors cause these abnormalities.

Cleft Hand or Foot (Fig. 16-9*E* and *F*). In this rare deformity, often called the lobster-claw deformity, there is absence of one or more central digits. Thus the hand or foot is divided into two parts that oppose each other like lobster claws. The remaining digits are partially or completely fused (syndactyly).

Brachydactyly (Fig. 16-10*A*). Abnormal

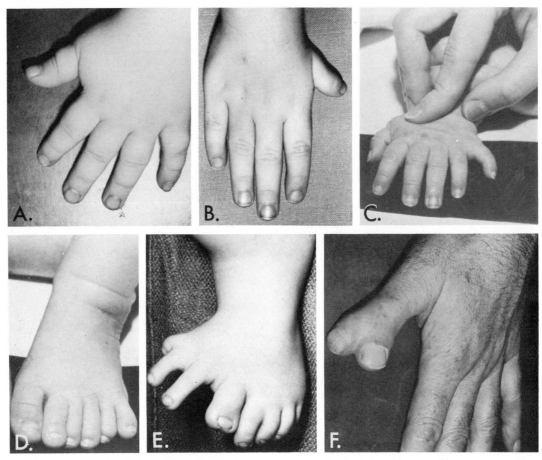

Figure 16–10. Photographs of various types of limb deformities. *A*, Brachydactyly. *B*, Hypoplasia (under-development) of the thumb. *C*, Polydactyly showing a supernumerary finger. *D*, Polydactyly showing a super-numerary toe. *E*, Partial duplication of the foot. *F*, Partial duplication of the thumb. (*C* and *D* are from Swenson, O.: *Pediatric Surgery*. 1958. Courtesy of Appleton-Century-Crofts, Inc.)

shortness of the fingers or toes is uncommon. This results from reduction in the size of the phalanges. It is usually inherited as a dominant trait and is often associated with shortness of stature.

Polydactyly or Supernumerary Digits (Fig. 16–10*C* and *D*). Supernumerary (extra) fingers or toes are common. Often the extra digit is incompletely formed and is useless. If the hand is affected, the extra digit is most commonly ulnar or radial in position rather than central. In the foot, the extra toe is usually in the fibular position. Polydactyly is inherited as a dominant trait.

Syndactyly or Webbed Digits (Fig. 16–11). Fusion of the fingers or toes is a common limb malformation. Webbing of the skin between the fingers or toes results from failure of the tissue to break down between the digits during development (Fig. 16–4*E* and *K*). Syndactyly is most frequently observed between third and fourth fingers and the second and third toes. It is inherited as a simple dominant or simple recessive trait.

Clubfoot or Talipes Equinovarus (Fig. 16–11*C*). This type of clubfoot is relatively common and is about twice as frequent in males. The sole of the foot is turned medially and the foot is adducted and plantar-flexed at the midtarsal joint. Although it is commonly stated that this condition results from abnormal positioning or restricted movement of the lower extremities *in utero*, the evidence for this is inconclusive. Hereditary and environmental factors appear to be involved in most cases.

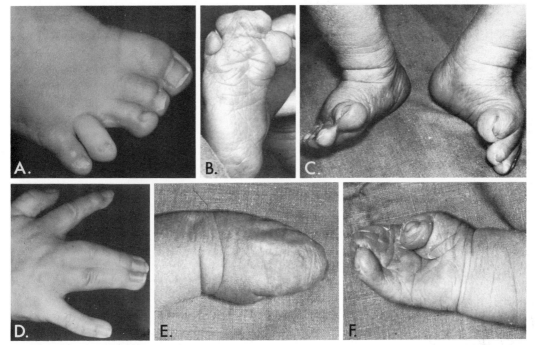

Figure 16-11. Photographs of various types of limb deformities. *A*, Syndactyly showing skin webs between the first and second and second and third toes. *B*, Syndactyly involving fusion of all the toes except the fifth. *C*, Syndactyly associated with clubfoot or talipes equinovarus. *D*, Syndactyly involving webbing of the third and fourth fingers. *E* and *F*, Dorsal and palmar views of a child's right hand showing syndactyly or fusion of the second to fifth fingers. (*A* and *D* are from Swenson, O.: *Pediatric Surgery*. 1958. Courtesy of Appleton-Century-Crofts, Inc.)

SUMMARY

The skeletal and muscular systems are derived from mesoderm. The skeleton mainly develops from condensed mesenchyme which undergoes chondrification to form hyaline cartilage models of the bones. Ossification centers appear in these models by the end of the embryonic period. Some bones develop by intramembranous ossification. The vertebral column and ribs develop from cells that originate in the somites. The developing skull consists of a neurocranium and a viscerocranium, each of which has membranous and cartilaginous components.

The limb buds appear during the fourth week as slight elevations of the ventrolateral body wall. The arm buds develop slightly before the leg buds. The tissues of the limb buds are derived from two main sources, the somatic mesoderm of the lateral plate and the ectoderm. The upper and lower limbs rotate in opposite directions and to different degrees.

Most skeletal muscle is derived from the myotome regions of the somites, but some head and neck muscles are derived from branchial arch mesoderm, and the limb musculature develops from mesenchyme derived from the somatic mesoderm. Cardiac and smooth muscle are derived from splanchnic mesoderm.

The majority of malformations of the skeletal and muscular systems are caused by genetic factors; however, many deformities probably result from an interaction of genetic and environmental factors.

17

THE NERVOUS
SYSTEM

The nervous system develops from the *neural plate*, a thickened area of embryonic ectoderm which appears during the third week. Formation of the *neural tube* and *neural crest* from the neural plate is illustrated in Figure 17–1. The neural tube differentiates into the *central nervous system*, consisting of the brain and spinal cord; the neural crest gives rise to most of the *peripheral nervous system*.

THE CENTRAL NERVOUS SYSTEM

The neural tube is temporarily open both cranially and caudally (Figs. 17–1*C* and 17–2*A* to *C*). These openings, called *neuropores*, close during the fourth week. The walls of the neural tube thicken to form the brain and the spinal cord (Fig. 17–3). The neural canal becomes the ventricles of the brain and the central canal of the spinal cord.

THE SPINAL CORD

The lateral walls of the neural tube thicken until only a small *central canal* remains (Fig. 17–4*C*). The wall of the neural tube is composed of a thick neuroepithelium which gives rise to all neurons and macroglial cells of the spinal cord (Fig. 17–5). The marginal zone of the neuroepithelium gradually becomes the white matter of the cord as axons grow into it from nerve cell bodies in the spinal cord, in the dorsal root ganglia and in the brain.

Some neuroepithelial cells differentiate into immature neurons called *neuroblasts*. These cells form an *intermediate zone* between the ventricular and marginal zones (Fig. 17–4*E*). When the neuroepithelial cells cease producing neuroblasts and glioblasts, they differentiate into ependymal cells which give rise to the ependymal epithelium (ependyma) lining the central canal of the spinal cord.

The *microglial cells* (microglia), a smaller type of neuroglial cell, differentiate from mesenchymal cells surrounding the central nervous system (Fig. 17–5). They enter the spinal cord with developing blood vessels.

Thickening of the lateral walls of the spinal cord soon produces a shallow longitudinal groove called the *sulcus limitans* (Figs. 17–4*B* and 17–6). This groove demarcates the dorsal part or *alar plate* (lamina) from the ventral part or *basal plate* (lamina). The alar and basal plates are later associated with afferent and efferent functions respectively.

The Alar Plates. Cell bodies in the alar plates form the dorsal horns (Fig. 17–7). As these plates enlarge, the *dorsal septum* forms and the central canal becomes small (Figs. 17–4*C* and 17–7).

The Basal Plates. Cell bodies in the basal plates form the ventral and lateral horns. Axons of ventral horn cells grow out of the spinal cord and form large bundles called *anterior (ventral) roots* of the spinal nerves (Fig. 17–6). As the basal plates enlarge, they produce the *ventral median septum* and a deep longitudinal groove on the ventral surface of the spinal cord known as the *ventral median fissure* (Figs. 17–4*C* and 17–7).

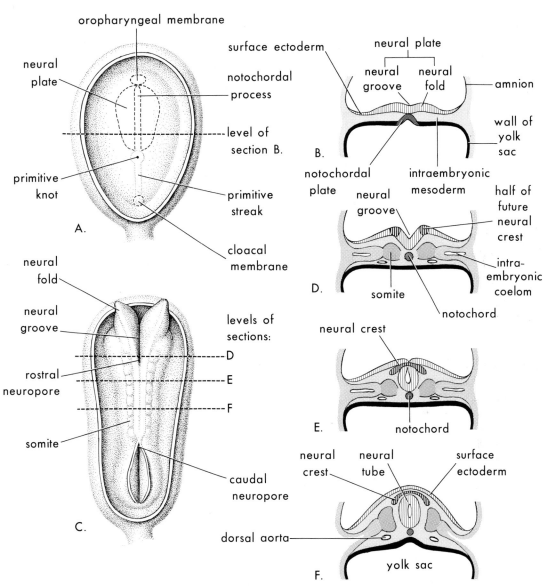

Figure 17-1. Diagrams illustrating formation of the neural crest and folding of the neural plate into the neural tube. *A,* Dorsal view of an embryo of about 18 days, exposed by removing the amnion. *B,* Transverse section of this embryo showing the neural plate and early development of the neural groove. *C,* Dorsal view of an embryo of about 22 days. The neural folds have fused opposite the somites, but are widely spread out at both ends of the embryo. *D, E* and *F,* Transverse sections of this embryo at the levels shown in *C,* illustrating formation of the neural tube and its detachment from the surface ectoderm. Note that some neuroectodermal cells are not included in the neural tube but remain between it and the surface ectoderm as the neural crest.

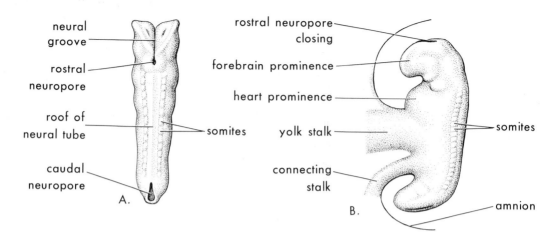

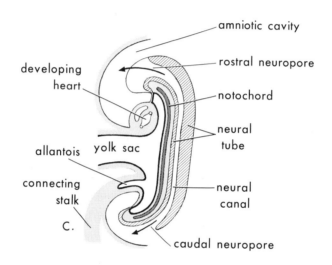

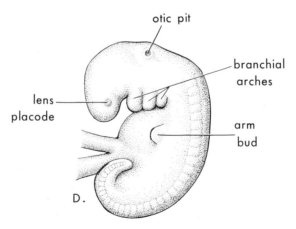

Figure 17–2. *A*, Dorsal view of an embryo of about 23 days showing advanced fusion of the neural folds. *B*, Lateral view of an embryo of about 24 days showing the forebrain prominence and closing of the rostral neuropore. *C*, Sagittal section of this embryo showing the transitory communication of the neural canal with the amniotic cavity (arrows). *D*, Lateral view of an embryo of 26 days after closure of the neuropores.

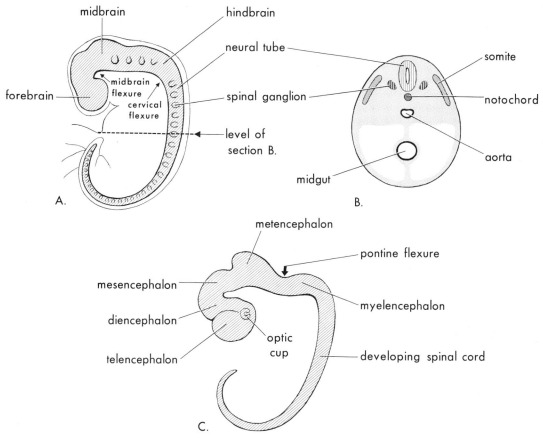

Figure 17–3. *A,* Schematic lateral view of an embryo of about 28 days showing the three primary brain vesicles. The two flexures demarcate the primary divisions of the brain. *B,* Transverse section of this embryo showing the neural tube which, in this region, will develop into the spinal cord. The spinal ganglia derived from the neural crest are also shown. *C,* Schematic lateral view of the central nervous system of a six-week embryo, showing the secondary brain vesicles and the pontine flexure.

Dorsal Root Ganglia. The unipolar neurons in the dorsal root ganglia (Figs. 17–6 and 17–7) are derived from neural crest cells. Their axons divide in a T-shaped fashion into central and peripheral processes. The central branches or processes enter the spinal cord and constitute the *dorsal (posterior) roots* of spinal nerves (Fig. 17–7). The peripheral processes of dorsal root ganglion cells pass in the spinal nerves (Fig. 17–6) to special sensory endings in somatic or visceral structures.

Positional Changes of the Spinal Cord. The spinal cord initially extends the entire length of the vertebral canal, and the spinal nerves pass through the intervertebral foramina at their levels of origin (Fig. 17–8A). This relationship does not persist because

the vertebral column and the dura mater (outer covering of the spinal cord) grow more rapidly than the spinal cord. The caudal end of the spinal cord gradually comes to lie at relatively higher levels. As a result, the spinal roots, especially those of the lumbar and sacral segments, run obliquely from the spinal cord to the corresponding level of the vertebral column. The dorsal and ventral nerve roots below the end of the cord form a sheaf of nerve roots called the *cauda equina* (Fig. 17–8D). Although the dura extends the entire length of the vertebral column in the adult, the other layers of the meninges do not. The pia mater beyond the caudal end of the spinal cord forms a long fibrous thread, the *filum terminale,* which extends from the conus

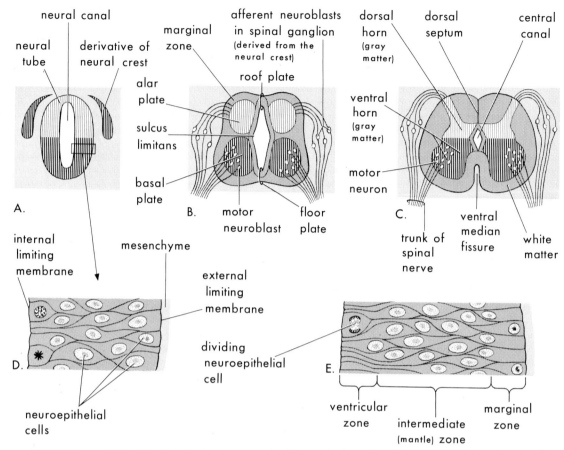

Figure 17–4. Diagrams illustrating development of the spinal cord. *A,* Transverse section through the neural tube of an embryo of about 23 days. *B* and *C,* Similar sections at six and nine weeks, respectively. *D,* Section through the wall of the early neural tube. *E,* Section through the wall of the developing spinal cord showing the three different zones.

medullaris (conical extremity of the spinal cord) and attaches to the periosteum of the first coccygeal vertebra in the adult. A portion of the subarachnoid space extends below the spinal cord (usually from L_1 to L_3) from which cerebrospinal fluid may be removed without damaging the cord. The removal of cerebrospinal fluid by insertion of a needle between certain lumbar vertebrae and into the subarachnoid space is known as *lumbar puncture.*

Myelination. Myelin formation begins in the spinal cord during midfetal life and continues during the first postnatal year. The myelin sheath is formed around axons or axis cylinders by the plasma membranes of *Schwann cells* (Fig. 17–9*A* to *E*). The myelin sheath of axons in the central nervous sys-

tem is formed in a somewhat similar manner by *oligodendrocytes* (Fig. 17–9*F* to *H*).

THE BRAIN

Brain Vesicles. During the fourth week, the neural folds expand and fuse to form three primary brain vesicles: the *forebrain* or prosencephalon, the *midbrain* or mesencephalon, and the *hindbrain* or rhombencephalon (Figs. 17–3*A* and 17–10). During the fifth week, the forebrain partly divides into two vesicles, the *telencephalon* and the *diencephalon,* and the hindbrain partly divides into the *metencephalon* and the *myelencephalon.* As a result, there are five secondary brain vesicles.

(Text continued on page 204.)

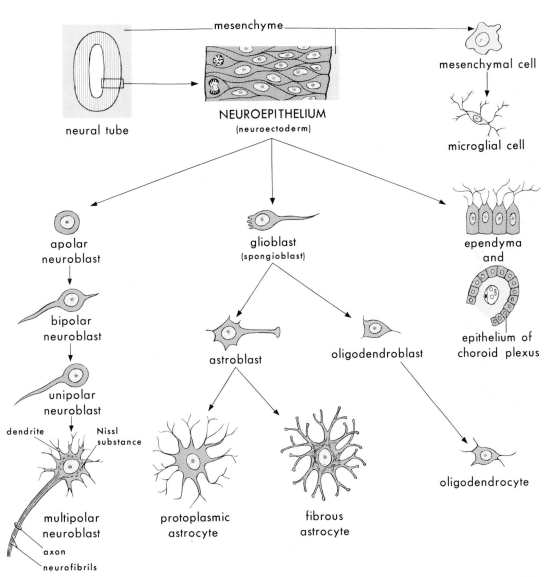

Figure 17–5. Schematic diagram illustrating the histogenesis of cells in the central nervous system. With further development, the multipolar neuroblast (lower left) becomes a nerve cell or neuron. Neuroepithelial cells give rise to all neurons and macroglial cells. Microglial cells are derived from mesenchymal cells which invade the developing nervous system.

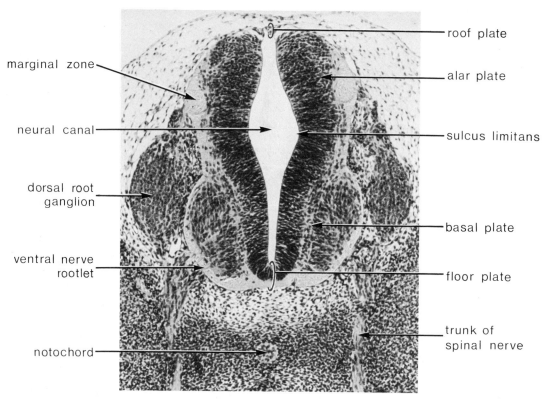

marginal zone

neural canal

dorsal root ganglion

ventral nerve rootlet

notochord

roof plate

alar plate

sulcus limitans

basal plate

floor plate

trunk of spinal nerve

Figure 17-6. Photomicrograph of a transverse section of the developing spinal cord in a 14-mm human embryo of about 36 days (×75). The dorsal wall (roof plate) and the ventral wall (floor plate) contain no neuroblasts and are relatively thin. (Courtesy of Dr. J. W. A. Duckworth, Professor of Anatomy, University of Toronto.)

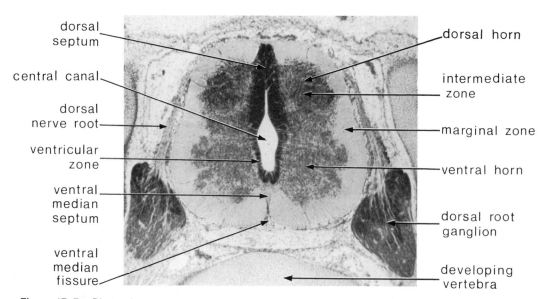

dorsal septum

central canal

dorsal nerve root

ventricular zone

ventral median septum

ventral median fissure

dorsal horn

intermediate zone

marginal zone

ventral horn

dorsal root ganglion

developing vertebra

Figure 17-7. Photomicrograph of a transverse section of the developing spinal cord in a 20-mm human embryo of about 40 days (×60).

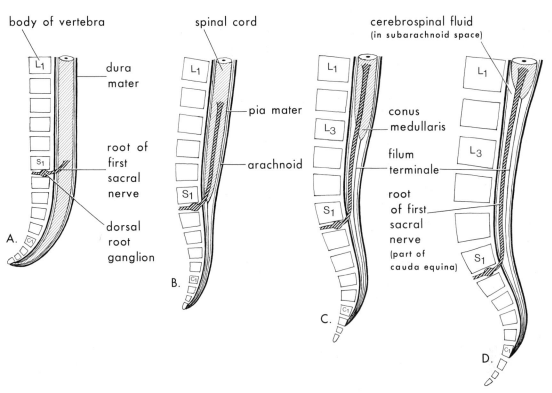

Figure 17-8. Diagrams showing the position of the caudal end of the spinal cord in relation to the vertebral column and the meninges at various stages of development. The increasing inclination of the root of the first sacral nerve is also illustrated. *A*, Eight weeks. *B*, 24 weeks. *C*, Newborn. *D*, Adult.

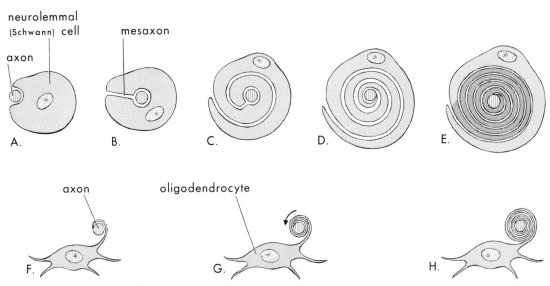

Figure 17-9. Diagrammatic sketches illustrating myelination of axons. *A* to *E*, Successive stages in the myelination of a peripheral nerve fiber or axon by a Schwann cell. The axon first indents the cell, then the Schwann cell apparently rotates around the axon as the mesaxon (site of invagination) elongates. The cytoplasm between the layers of cell membrane gradually condenses. Cytoplasm remains on the inside of the sheath between the myelin and axon. *F* to *H*, Successive stages in the myelination of a nerve fiber in the central nervous system by an oligodendrocyte. A process of the neuroglial cell wraps itself around the axon, and the intervening layers of cytoplasm move to the body of the cell.

3 PRIMARY
VESICLES

5 SECONDARY   ADULT DERIVATIVES
VESICLES   OF
                    WALLS   CAVITIES

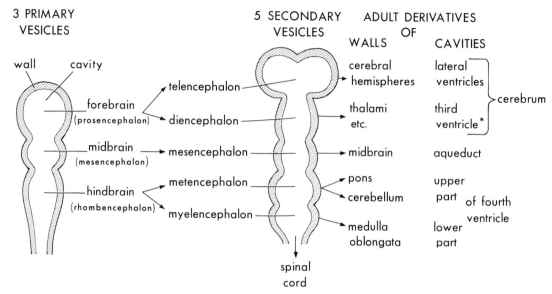

Figure 17–10. Diagrammatic sketches of the brain vesicles indicating the adult derivatives of their walls and cavities. The cerebrum comprises all the derivatives of the forebrain. *The extreme anterior part of the third ventricle forms from the cavity of the telencephalon.

Brain Flexures. During the fourth week the brain grows rapidly and bends or flexes ventrally (Fig. 17–3). This produces the *midbrain flexure* in the midbrain region and the *cervical flexure* at the junction of the hindbrain and the spinal cord. Later, unequal growth in the hindbrain produces the *pontine flexure* between these flexures; this flexure causes thinning of the roof of the hindbrain (Fig. 17–11*A* and *C*).

Initially, the developing brain has the same basic structure as the early spinal cord; however, the brain flexures produce considerable variation in the outline of transverse sections at different levels of the brain and in the position of the gray and white matter.

The Hindbrain

The cervical flexure demarcates the hindbrain vesicle from the developing spinal cord (Fig. 17–11*A*). The pontine flexure appears in the future pontine region. The bend of this flexure divides the hindbrain into caudal (myelencephalon) and rostral (metencephalon) parts. The myelencephalon becomes the *medulla oblongata*, and the metencephalon gives rise to the *pons* and *cerebellum*. The cavity of the hindbrain becomes the fourth ventricle and the central canal of the lower medulla.

The Myelencephalon (Fig. 17–11). The caudal part of the myelencephalon resembles the spinal cord. The lumen of the neural tube becomes a small central canal. Unlike the spinal cord, neuroblasts from the alar plates migrate into the marginal zone and form the *gracile nucleus* medially and the *cuneate nucleus* laterally (Fig. 17–11*B*). The ventral area contains a pair of fiber bundles, called the *pyramids*, consisting of nerve fibers from the developing cerebral cortex.

The rostral part of the myelencephalon (the developing "open" portion of the medulla) is wide and rather flat, especially opposite the pontine flexure (Fig. 17–11*A* and *C*). The pontine flexure causes the lateral walls of the medulla to fall outward like the pages of an opening book and the roof plate to become stretched.

The Metencephalon (Fig. 17–12). The walls of the metencephalon form the pons and the cerebellum, and its cavity forms the upper part of the fourth ventricle. As in the rostral part of the myelencephalon, the pontine flexure causes divergence of the lateral walls of the medulla and spreads the gray matter in the floor of the fourth ventricle.

The *cerebellum* develops from thickenings of dorsal parts of the alar plates which enlarge and fuse in the midline. These cerebellar swellings soon overgrow the rostral half of the fourth ventricle and overlap the pons and medulla (Fig. 17–12*D*).

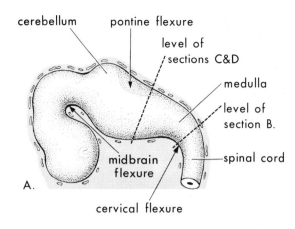

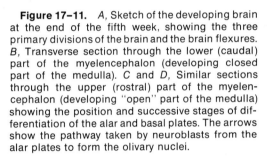

Figure 17–11. *A*, Sketch of the developing brain at the end of the fifth week, showing the three primary divisions of the brain and the brain flexures. *B*, Transverse section through the lower (caudal) part of the myelencephalon (developing closed part of the medulla). *C* and *D*, Similar sections through the upper (rostral) part of the myelencephalon (developing "open" part of the medulla) showing the position and successive stages of differentiation of the alar and basal plates. The arrows show the pathway taken by neuroblasts from the alar plates to form the olivary nuclei.

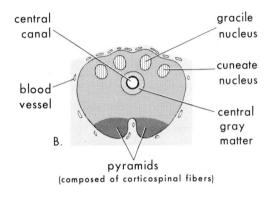

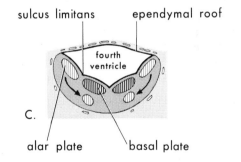

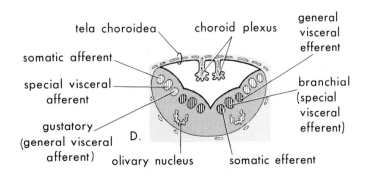

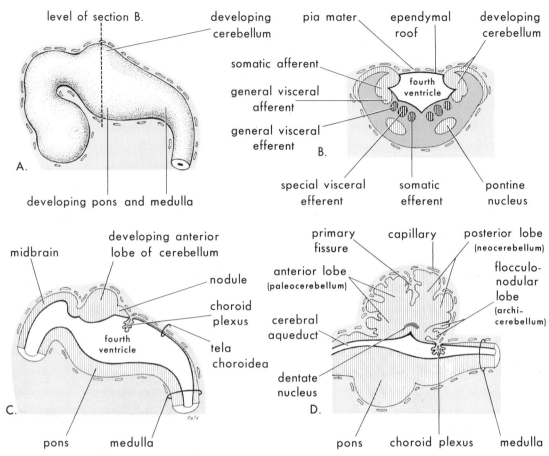

Figure 17–12. *A*, Sketch of the developing brain at the end of the fifth week. *B*, Transverse section through the metencephalon (developing pons and cerebellum) showing the derivatives of the alar and basal plates. *C* and *D*, Sagittal sections of the hindbrain at about six and 17 weeks, respectively, showing successive stages of development of the pons and cerebellum.

Nerve fibers connecting the cerebral and cerebellar cortices with the spinal cord pass through the marginal layer of the ventral region of the metencephalon. This region of the brainstem is called the *pons* (from Latin, meaning "bridge"), because of the band of nerve fibers thus formed.

Choroid Plexuses and Cerebrospinal Fluid (Figs. 17–11*D* and 17–12*C* and *D*). The thin ependymal roof of the fourth ventricle is covered externally by vascular *pia mater*. This pia mater together with the ependymal roof forms the *tela choroidea* which invaginates into the fourth ventricle and forms the choroid plexus. Similar plexuses develop in the roof of the third ventricle and in the medial walls of the lateral ventricles. Four choroid plexuses are formed and are responsible for the secretion of cerebrospinal fluid. The thin roof of the fourth ventricle bulges outward in three locations and ruptures to form foramina. The median and lateral apertures permit the cerebrospinal fluid from the fourth ventricle to enter the *subarachnoid space* (Fig. 17–8*D*).

The Midbrain

The midbrain undergoes less change than any part of the developing brain, except the lower part of the hindbrain. The neural canal narrows to form the cerebral aqueduct (Figs. 17–12*D* and 17–13*D*), which joins the third and fourth ventricles. Neuroblasts migrate from the alar plates into the roof or *tectum* and aggregate to form four large groups of neurons, the paired *superior* and

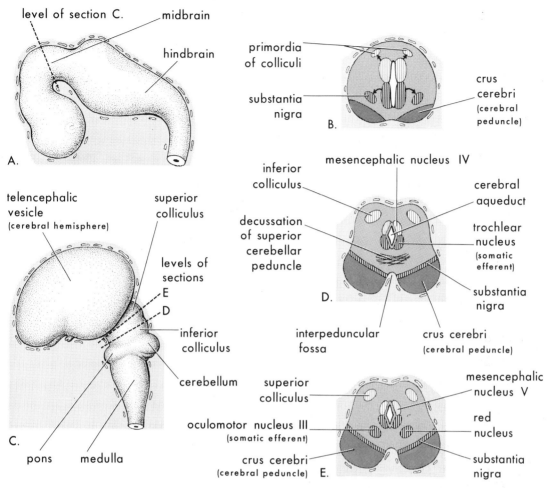

Figure 17–13. *A*, Sketch of the developing brain at the end of the fifth week. *B*, Transverse section through the mesencephalon (developing midbrain) showing basal and alar plates. *C*, Sketch of the developing brain at about 11 weeks. *D* and *E*, Transverse sections of the developing midbrain at the level of the inferior and superior colliculi, respectively.

inferior colliculi (concerned with visual and auditory reflexes respectively). The basal plates give rise to neurons of the *tegmentum* (red nuclei, nuclei of the third and fourth cranial nerves and neurons of the reticular nuclei). Fibers growing from the cerebrum form the cerebral peduncles. The *substantia nigra* (black nucleus), a broad layer of gray matter adjacent to the cerebral peduncle, differentiates from the basal plate.

The Forebrain

The forebrain has a central part, the *diencephalon* or intermediate brain, and lateral expansions, the right and left cerebral vesi-cles or *telencephalon* (endbrain). The forebrain develops into the cerebrum, and its cavity forms the slit-like third ventricle.

The Diencephalon (Fig. 17–14). Three swellings develop in the lateral walls of the third ventricle; these later become the *epithalamus*, the *thalamus* and the *hypothalamus*. The *thalamus* on each side develops rapidly and bulges into the cavity of the third ventricle, reducing it to a narrow cleft. The *hypothalamus* arises by proliferation of neuroblasts in the intermediate zone of the diencephalic walls below the hypothalamic sulcus (Fig. 17–14). The *pineal gland* (epiphysis) develops as a midline diverticulum of the caudal part of the diencephalic roof (Fig. 17–14*D*).

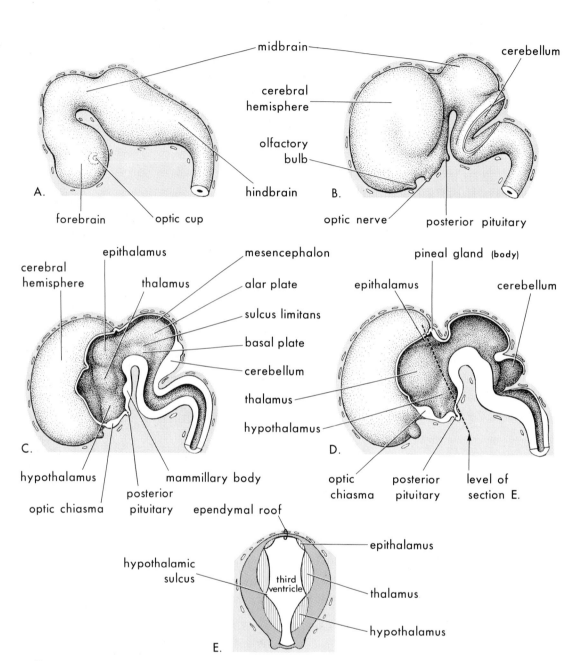

Figure 17–14. *A,* External view of the brain at the end of the fifth week. *B,* Similar view at seven weeks. *C,* Median sagittal section of this brain showing the medial surface of the forebrain and midbrain. *D,* Similar section at eight weeks. *E,* Transverse section through the diencephalon showing the epithalamus dorsally, the thalamus laterally and the hypothalamus ventrally.

The Telencephalon (Fig. 17–15). The telencephalon consists of a median part and two cerebral vesicles. The cavity of the median portion forms the extreme anterior part of the third ventricle. At first the cerebral vesicles are in wide communication with the cavity of the third ventricle through the *interventricular foramina* (Fig. 17–16*B*). As the hemispheres expand, somewhat like inflating balloons, they cover the diencephalon, the midbrain and the hindbrain. The hemispheres eventually meet each other in the midline, flattening their medial surfaces.

The *corpus striatum* appears as a prominent swelling in the floor of each hemisphere (Fig. 17–16*B*). The floor of the hemisphere expands more slowly than the thin cortical wall because it contains the rather large corpus striatum. Consequently, the cerebral hemispheres assume a C-shape (Fig. 17–15). Backward extension of the hemispheres is limited, thus its caudal end turns downward and forward, forming the temporal lobe.

As the cerebral cortex differentiates, fibers passing to and from it through the corpus striatum divide it into *caudate* and *lentiform nuclei*. This important fiber pathway is called the *internal capsule* (Fig. 17–16*C*).

The Cerebral Cortex. The walls of the developing cerebral hemispheres initially show the typical zones of the neural tube. Cells of the intermediate zone migrate into the marginal zone and give rise to the cortical layers. Thus, the gray matter is located marginally, and axons from its cell bodies pass centrally and not peripherally as in the spinal cord.

Initially the surface of the hemispheres is smooth (Fig. 17–15*A*), but as growth proceeds, sulci and gyri develop. These permit increase in the volume of the cerebral cortex without requiring an extensive increase in cranial volume.

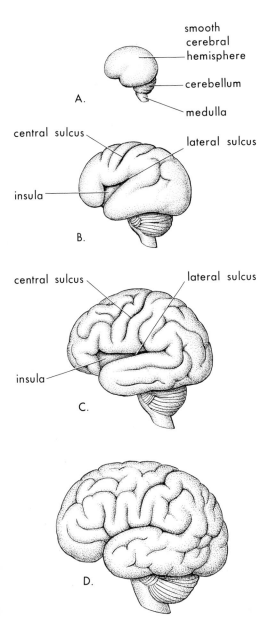

Figure 17–15. Sketches of lateral views of the left cerebral hemisphere showing successive stages in the development of sulci and gyri. *Half actual size.* Note the gradual narrowing of the lateral sulcus and formation of the insula. *A,* 13 weeks. *B,* 26 weeks. *C,* 35 weeks. *D,* Newborn.

The Pituitary Gland

This gland develops from two sources: ectoderm of the primitive mouth cavity and neuroectoderm of the diencephalon (Fig. 17–17 and Table 17–1). This double origin explains why the pituitary is composed of two completely different types of tissue. The *adenohypophysis* (glandular portion) arises from the oral ectoderm, and the neurohypophysis (nervous portion) originates from the neuroectoderm.

During the third week, a diverticulum called *Rathke's pouch* arises from the roof of the primitive mouth cavity and grows toward the brain. This pouch elongates and comes into contact with the *infundibulum,*

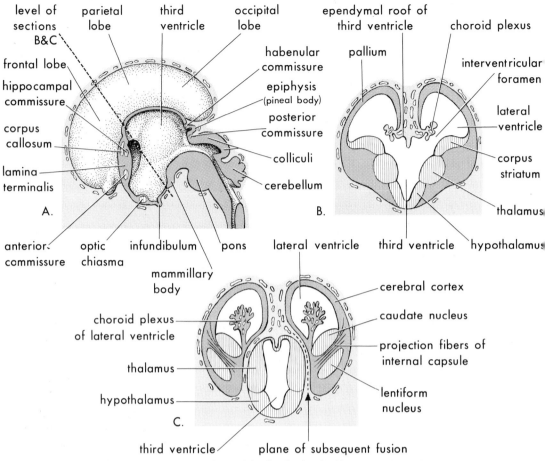

Figure 17–16. *A,* Drawing of medial surface of the forebrain of a 10-week embryo showing the diencephalic derivatives, the main commissures and the expanding telencephalic (cerebral) vesicle. *B,* Transverse section through the forebrain at the level of the interventricular foramen showing the corpus striatum and the choroid plexus of the lateral ventricle. *C,* Similar section at about 11 weeks showing division of the corpus striatum into caudate and lentiform nuclei by the internal capsule.

which develops as a ventral diverticulum of the floor of the diencephalon (Fig. 17–17*B*).

Adenohypophysis. Early during the sixth week, the connection of Rathke's pouch with the oral cavity disappears (Fig. 17–17*D* and *E*). Cells of the anterior wall of Rathke's pouch proliferate actively and give rise to the *pars distalis* of the pituitary gland. Later a small extension, the *pars tuberalis*, extends around the *infundibular stem.* Proliferation of the anterior wall of Rathke's pouch reduces the lumen to a narrow residual cleft (Fig. 17–17*E*). The posterior wall does not proliferate; it remains as the poorly defined *pars intermedia* which is composed of a thin layer of cells and vesicles.

Neurohypophysis. The small infundibulum gives rise to the *median eminence,* the *in-*

fundibular stem and the *pars nervosa* (Fig. 17–17*F*). Nerve fibers grow into the pars nervosa from the hypothalamic area to which the infundibular stem is attached.

THE PERIPHERAL NERVOUS SYSTEM

The peripheral nervous system consists of the cranial, spinal and visceral nerves and the cranial, spinal and autonomic ganglia. Afferent neurons in the dorsal root ganglia and ganglia of cranial nerves develop from *neural crest cells* (Figs. 17–1 and 17–18). Cells of the neural crest also differentiate into multipolar neurons of the *autonomic ganglia,*

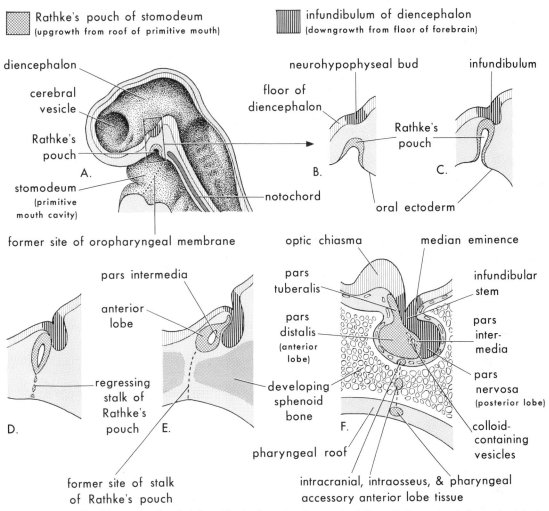

Rathke's pouch of stomodeum
(upgrowth from roof of primitive mouth)

infundibulum of diencephalon
(downgrowth from floor of forebrain)

Figure 17–17. Diagrammatic sketches illustrating development of the pituitary gland (hypophysis). *A,* Sagittal section of the cranial end of an embryo at four weeks showing Rathke's pouch as an upgrowth from the roof of the primitive mouth cavity, and the neurohypophyseal bud from the forebrain. *B to D,* Successive stages of the developing pituitary gland. By eight weeks, Rathke's pouch loses its connection with the oral cavity, *E and F,* Later stages, showing proliferation of the anterior wall of Rathke's pouch and obliteration of its lumen.

including ganglia of the sympathetic trunks along the sides of the vertebral bodies, collateral or prevertebral ganglia in plexuses of the thorax and abdomen (e.g., the cardiac, celiac and mesenteric plexuses), and para-sympathetic or terminal ganglia in or near the viscera (e.g., the Meissner's or submucosal plexus). *Chromaffin cells* of the paraganglia are also derived from the neural crest. The carotid and aortic bodies also

TABLE 17–1. DERIVATION AND TERMINOLOGY OF THE PITUITARY GLAND

Oral Ectoderm
(From roof of primitive mouth [stomodeum]) ⟶ Adenohypophysis (glandular portion) — Pars distalis, Pars tuberalis — Anterior lobe; Pars intermedia — Posterior lobe

Neuroectoderm
(From floor of diencephalon) ⟶ Neurohypophysis (nervous portion) — Pars nervosa, Infundibular stem, Median eminence — Posterior lobe

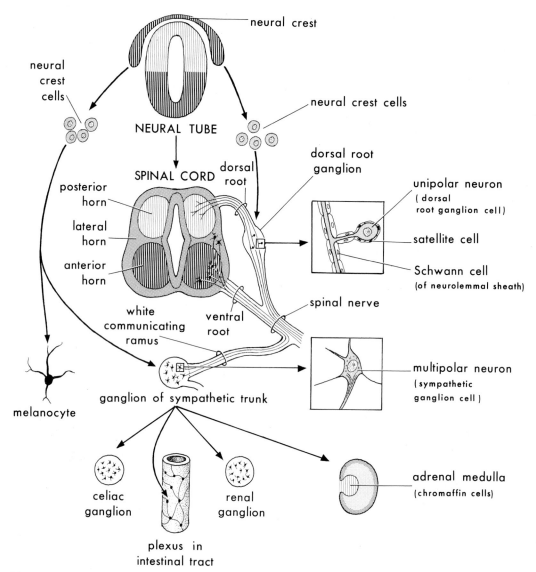

Figure 17–18. Diagram showing the derivatives of neural crest cells. Neural crest cells also differentiate into cells of the afferent ganglia of cranial nerves. Formation of a spinal nerve is also illustrated.

have small islands of chromaffin cells associated with them. These widely scattered groups of chromaffin cells constitute the *chromaffin system.*

CONGENITAL MALFORMATIONS OF THE NERVOUS SYSTEM

Most major congenital malformations result from defective formation of the neural tube during the third and fourth weeks. These abnormalities may be limited to the nervous system, or they may involve overlying tissues (bone, muscle and connective tissue). Some malformations are caused by genetic abnormalities, and some result from environmental factors such as infectious agents, drugs and ionizing radiation. Most severe abnormalities of the central nervous system are incompatible with survival; less severe malformations cause functional disability. It is well established that abnormalities of the central nervous system may result from fetal infection with *Toxoplasma gondii.*

Spina Bifida. Various types of malformation of the central nervous system are associated with defective fusion of structures dorsal to the spinal cord. The term spina bifida refers to a defect of the vertebral column (Chapter 16). Clinically, it is commonly used in reference to conditions involving both vertebral and neural defects. Spina bifida is most common in the lower thoracic, lumbar and sacral regions.

Spina Bifida Occulta (Fig. 17–19*A*). This common and least serious type of spina bifida is discussed in Chapter 16. The defect is covered by skin, and often a small tuft of hair, an area of pigmentation or both appear over the defect. Usually there are no neurological or musculoskeletal disturbances associated with spina bifida occulta.

Spina Bifida Cystica (Figs. 17–19*B* to *D* and 17–20) is a severe type of spina bifida. There is an external protrusion of the meninges or spinal cord and meninges through the defective vertebrae. When the sac contains only meninges and cerebrospinal fluid, the condition is called *spina bifida with meningocele* (Fig. 17–19*B*). If the spinal cord and spinal roots or the cauda equina are included in the sac, the malformation is called *spina bifida with meningomyelocele* (Figs. 17–19*C* and 17–20). This abnormality is a commoner and very much more severe malformation than meningocele. The incidence of meningomyeloceles is slightly more than one per thousand live births.

Spina bifida cystica shows varying degrees

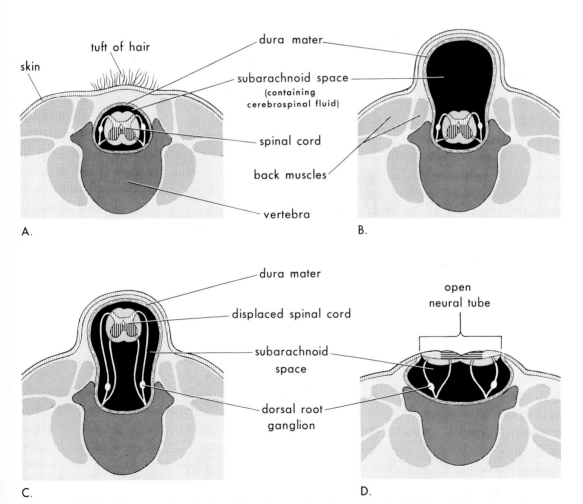

Figure 17–19. Diagrammatic sketches illustrating various types of spina bifida and the commonly associated malformations of the nervous system. *A,* Spina bifida occulta. *B,* Spina bifida with meningocele. *C,* Spina bifida with meningomyelocele. *B,* Spina bifida with myeloschisis. (Modified after Patten, 1968.)

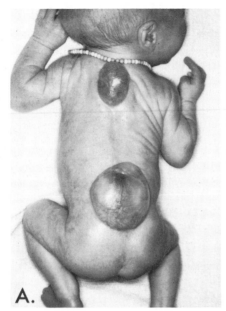
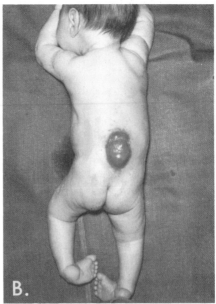

Figure 17–20. Photographs of infants with spina bifida cystica showing the common locations of these defects. *A*, Spina bifida with meningomyelocele in the thoracic and lumbar regions. *B*, Spina bifida with myeloschisis in the lumbar region. Note the nerve involvement affecting the lower extremities. (Courtesy of Dr. Dwight Parkinson, Children's Centre, Winnipeg.)

of neurological involvement depending on the position and extent of the lesion. There is usually a corresponding loss of sensation along with complete or partial skeletal muscle paralysis (Fig. 17–20*B*). The level of the lesion determines the area of anesthesia and which muscles are affected.

Anencephaly (Fig. 16–7). Anencephaly is a common malformation (one per thousand births). Sustained extrauterine life is impossible. Although the term anencephaly means absence of the brain, there is always some brain tissue present in anencephalic infants. Animal experiments show that anencephaly results from failure of the neural folds in the cranial end of the neural plate to fuse and form the forebrain. Genetic factors are certainly involved because of the well-established familial incidence of anencephaly. An excess of amniotic fluid (polyhydramnios, Chapter 8) is often associated with anencephaly.

Microcephaly (Fig. 17–21). In this uncommon condition, the cranium is small but the face is normal-sized. These infants are generally grossly retarded mentally. The cause of this condition is often uncertain; some cases appear to be genetic in origin, and others seem to be associated with environmental factors. X-ray exposure during the embryonic period and infectious agents

during the fetal period are possible contributing factors (see Chapter 9).

Cranial Encephalocele and Meningocele

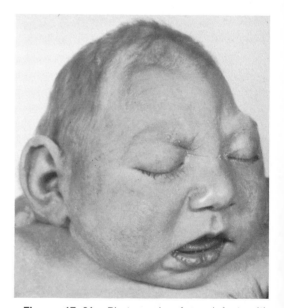

Figure 17–21. Photograph of an infant with microcephaly showing the typical normal-sized face and small cranial vault covered with loose wrinkled skin (From Laurence, K. M. and Weeks, R.: Abnormalities of the central nervous system; *in* A. P. Norman (Ed.): *Congenital Abnormalities in Infancy*, 2nd ed. 1971. Courtesy of Blackwell Scientific Publications.)

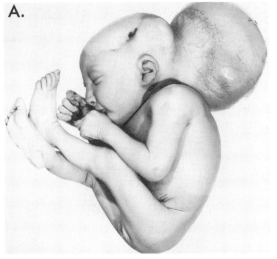 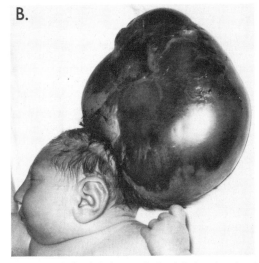

Figure 17-22. Photographs of infants with large encephaloceles. *A*, Occipital area. *B*, Occipital and parietal areas. (Courtesy of Dr. Dwight Parkinson, Children's Centre, Winnipeg.)

(Fig. 17-22). A portion of the brain and meninges herniates through a defect in the skull, usually in the occipital region. This condition occurs about once in 2000 births. Hydrocephalus (accumulation of cerebrospinal fluid) generally accompanies encephalocele. If the meningeal sac contains fluid only, it is called a cranial meningocele.

Hydrocephalus. Any abnormality characterized by accumulation of cerebrospinal fluid in the cranial vault is called hydrocephalus. Hydrocephalus may result from overproduction, failure of absorption or obstruction to the flow of cerebrospinal fluid. Hydrocephalus is often associated with spina bifida cystica, although the hydrocephalus may not be obvious at birth. Hydrocephalus often produces thinning of the bones of the cranial vault, prominence of the forehead and atrophy of the cerebral cortex.

Mental Retardation. Congenital impairment of intelligence may result from various genetically determined conditions. The relation of chromosomal abnormalities to mental retardation is briefly discussed in Chapter 9. Disorders of metabolism may also cause mental retardation. Maternal and fetal infections (syphilis, German measles, toxoplasmosis and cytomegalic inclusion disease), fetal irradiation and cretinism are commonly associated with mental retardation.

SUMMARY

The central nervous system develops from the *neural plate*. This plate becomes infolded to form a *neural groove* and *neural folds.* When the neural folds fuse to form the *neural tube,* some neuroectodermal cells are not included but remain between the neural tube and the surface ectoderm as the *neural crest.*

The cranial end of the neural tube forms the brain, consisting of the forebrain, the midbrain and the hindbrain. The forebrain gives rise to the cerebrum; the midbrain becomes the adult midbrain; and the hindbrain gives rise to the pons, cerebellum and medulla oblongata.

The remainder and longest part of the neural tube becomes the spinal cord. The lumen of the neural tube becomes the ventricles of the brain and the central canal of the spinal cord. The walls of the neural tube become thickened by proliferation of neuroepithelial cells which give rise to all nerve and macroglial cells in the central nervous system. The microglia are believed to differentiate from mesenchymal cells which enter the central nervous system with the blood vessels.

Cells in the cranial, spinal and autonomic ganglia are derived from the neural crest. *Schwann (neurilemmal) cells,* which myelinate the axons, also arise from the neural crest. Similarly, most of the autonomic nervous system and all chromaffin tissue, including the adrenal medulla, develop from the neural crest.

Congenital malformations of the central nervous system are common. Defects of closure of the neural tube account for most of these abnormalities. The defects may be limited to the nervous system, or they may include overlying tissues (bone, muscle and connective tissue). Some malformations are caused by genetic abnormalities; others result from such environmental factors as infectious agents, drugs, ionizing radiation and metabolic disease. However, most malformations are probably caused by an interaction of genetic and environmental factors. Gross abnormalities (e.g., anencephaly) are usually incompatible with life. Other severe malformations (e.g., spina bifida cystica) often cause functional disability (e.g., muscle paralysis). Mental retardation may result from chromosomal abnormalities, from metabolic disorders, maternal and fetal infections or irradiation occurring during prenatal life.

18

THE EYE AND
THE EAR

THE EYE

The eyes develop from three sources: neuroectoderm, surface ectoderm and mesoderm. Eye development is first evident early in the fourth week when a pair of *optic sulci* or *grooves* appears in the neural folds at the cranial end of the embryo (Fig. 18–1*A* and *B*). These grooves soon become a pair of hollow diverticula, called *optic vesicles*, which project from the sides of the forebrain (Fig. 18–1*C*). As these vesicles grow, their distal ends expand and their connections with the forebrain become constricted to form *optic stalks* (Fig. 18–1*D*). Concurrently, the surface ectoderm adjacent to the optic vesicles thickens and forms *lens placodes* (Fig. 18–1*C*). The central region of each lens placode rapidly invaginates, forming a *lens pit* (Fig. 18–1*D*). The edges of these pits gradually approach each other and fuse to form *lens vesicles* (Fig. 18–1*F*). Meanwhile the optic vesicles invaginate and become double-layered *optic cups*. The lens vesicles soon separate from the surface ectoderm and grooves, called *optic fissures*, develop on the inferior (caudal) surface of the optic cups and along the optic stalks (Fig. 18–1*E* to *H*). Blood vessels develop in the mesenchyme in these fissures. The *hyaloid artery* supplies the inner layer of the optic cup, the lens vesicle and the mesenchyme within optic cup, and the *hyaloid vein* returns blood from these structures. As the edges of the optic fissure come together and fuse, the hyaloid vessels are enclosed within the optic nerves (Fig. 18–2*E* and *F*). The distal portions of the hyaloid vessels eventually degenerate, but their proximal portions persist as the *central artery and vein of the retina*.

The Retina. The retina develops from the optic cup: the outer, thinner layer of the cup becomes the pigment epithelium and the inner, thicker layer differentiates into the neural layer of the retina. Because the optic vesicle is an outgrowth of the forebrain, the layers of the optic cup which form from the vesicle are continuous with the wall of the brain. Under the influence of the lens, the inner layer of the optic cup proliferates and forms a thick neuroepithelium. Subsequently, the cells of this layer differentiate into rods and cones, bipolar cells and ganglion cells. The neural layer of the developing retina is continuous with the inner layer of the optic stalk (Figs. 18–1*F* and *G* and 18–2*D*). Consequently, axons of the ganglion cells pass into the inner wall of the optic stalk and gradually convert it into the optic nerve (Fig. 18–2*B*, *D* and *F*).

The Ciliary Body. Because the pigmented portion of the epithelium of the ciliary body is derived from the outer layer of the optic cup, it is continuous with the pigment epithelium of the retina (Fig. 18–3). The nonpigmented portion of the ciliary epithelium represents the forward prolongation of the neural layer of the retina in which no neural elements differentiate. The ciliary muscle and connective tissue develop from mesenchyme at the edge of the optic cup.

The Iris. The iris is derived from the rim of the optic cup which partially covers the lens (Fig. 18–3*D*). The epithelium of the iris represents both layers of the optic cup and

217

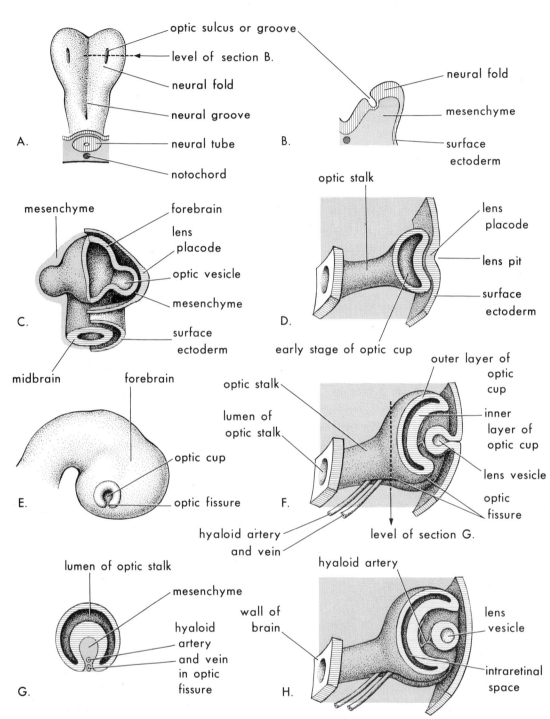

Figure 18–1. Drawings illustrating early eye development. A, Dorsal view of the cranial end of a 22-day embryo showing the first indication of eye development. B, Transverse section through an optic sulcus. C, Schematic drawing of the forebrain, its covering layers of mesoderm and surface ectoderm from an embryo of about 27 days. D, F and H, Schematic sections of the developing eye illustrating successive stages in the development of the optic cup and the lens vesicle. E, Lateral view of the brain of an embryo of about 28 days showing the external appearance of the optic cup. G, Transverse section through the optic stalk showing the optic fissure and its contents.

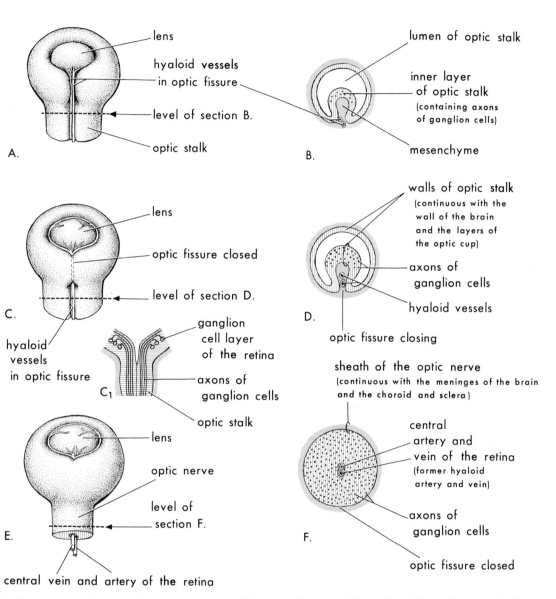

lens

hyaloid vessels
in optic fissure

level of section B.

optic stalk

A.

lumen of optic stalk

inner layer
of optic stalk
(containing axons
of ganglion cells)

mesenchyme

B.

lens

optic fissure closed

level of section D.

C.

hyaloid
vessels
in optic fissure

ganglion
cell layer
of the retina

axons of
ganglion cells

C_1

optic stalk

lens

optic nerve

level of
section F.

E.

central vein and artery of the retina

walls of optic stalk
(continuous with the
wall of the brain
and the layers of
the optic cup)

axons of
ganglion cells

hyaloid vessels

D.

optic fissure closing

sheath of the optic nerve
(continuous with the meninges of the brain
and the choroid and sclera)

central
artery and
vein of the retina
(former hyaloid
artery and vein)

axons of
ganglion cells

F.

optic fissure closed

Figure 18–2. Diagrams illustrating closure of the optic fissure and formation of the optic nerve. *A, C* and *E,* Views of the inferior surface of the optic cup and stalk showing progressive stages in the closure of the optic fissure. *C₁,* Schematic sketch of a longitudinal section of a portion of the optic cup and optic stalk showing axons of ganglion cells of the retina growing through the optic stalk to the brain. *B, D* and *F,* Transverse sections through the optic stalk showing successive stages in the closure of the optic fissure and in formation of the optic nerve. Note that the lumen of the optic stalk is gradually obliterated as axons of ganglion cells accumulate in the inner layer of the optic stalk.

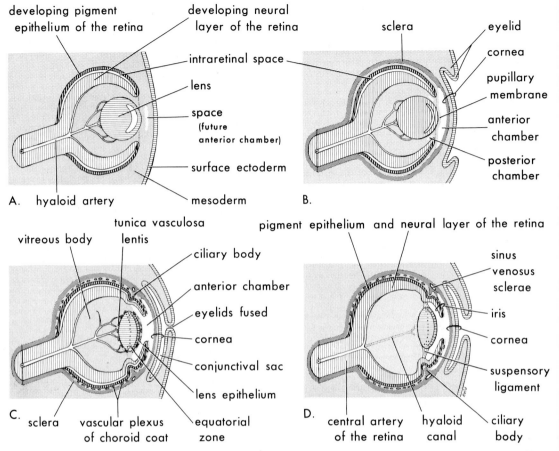

Figure 18–3. Drawings of sagittal sections of the eye showing successive developmental stages. *A*, Five weeks. *B*, Six weeks. *C*, 20 weeks. *D*, Newborn. Note that the layers of the optic cup are fused and form the pigment epithelium and neural layer of the retina and that they extend anteriorly as the double epithelium of the ciliary and iridial parts of the retina.

is continuous with the double-layered epithelium of the ciliary body and with the pigmented and neural layers of the retina. The dilator and sphincter pupillae muscles of the iris are derived from the neuroectoderm of the outer layer of the optic cup. The vascular connective tissue of the iris is derived from mesenchyme located anterior to the rim of the optic cup.

The Lens. The lens develops from the lens vesicle: the anterior wall becomes the anterior epithelium of the adult lens; cells of the posterior wall lengthen to form *lens fibers* which grow into and gradually obliterate the cavity of the lens vesicle (Fig. 18–3*A* to *C*). New lens fibers are continuously added to the lens from epithelial cells at the *equatorial zone* of the lens (Fig. 18–3*C*).

The Aqueous Chamber and the Cornea. The anterior chamber develops from a space which forms in the mesenchyme located between the developing lens and the surface ectoderm (Fig. 18–3*A* to *C*). The mesenchyme superficial to this space forms the substantia propria of the cornea. The epithelium of the cornea and the conjunctiva is derived from the surface ectoderm. The mesenchyme deep to the developing anterior chamber forms the stroma of the iris. The posterior chamber develops from a space which forms in the mesenchyme behind the developing iris and anterior to the developing lens (Fig. 18–3*B*).

The Sclera and Choroid. The mesenchyme surrounding the optic cup differentiates into an inner vascular layer, the choroid, and an outer fibrous layer, the sclera (Fig. 18–3*D*).

THE EAR

The Internal Ear. Early in the fourth week a thickened plate of surface ectoderm, the *otic placode*, appears on each side of the developing hindbrain (Fig. 18–4*A* and *B*). Each placode soon invaginates and forms an *otic pit* (Fig. 18–4*C* and *D*). The edges of the pit come together and fuse to form an otic vesicle or *otocyst*, the primordium of the *membranous labyrinth* (Fig. 18–4*E* to *G*). The otocyst soon loses its connection with the surface ectoderm.

Two regions of each otocyst soon become recognizable: a dorsal or *utricular portion* from which the endolymphatic duct arises,

and a ventral or *saccular portion*. Three flat disc-like diverticula grow out from the utricular portion, and soon the central portions of the walls of these diverticula fuse and then disappear (Fig. 18–5*B* to *E*). The peripheral unfused portions of the diverticula become the *semicircular canals*. From the ventral saccular portion of the otocyst, a tubular diverticulum, the *cochlear duct*, grows and coils to form the *cochlea* (Fig. 18–5*C* to *E*). The *organ of Corti* differentiates from cells in the wall of the cochlear duct (Fig. 18–5*F* to *T*).

The mesenchyme around the otocyst differentiates into a cartilaginous *otic capsule* (Fig. 18–5*F*). As the membranous labyrinth enlarges, vacuoles appear in the cartilaginous otic capsule and soon coalesce to form the *perilymphatic space*. The membranous labyrinth is soon suspended in a

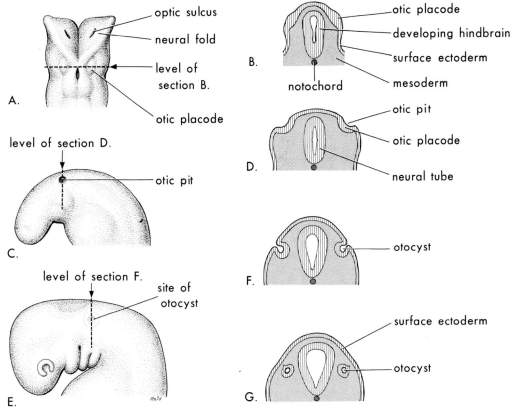

Figure 18–4. Drawings illustrating early development of the inner ear. *A,* Dorsal view of an embryo of about 22 days showing the otic placodes. *B, D, F* and *G,* Schematic sections illustrating successive stages in the development of the otocysts. *C* and *E,* Lateral views of the cranial region of embryos of about 24 and 28 days, respectively, showing the external appearance of the developing otocyst.

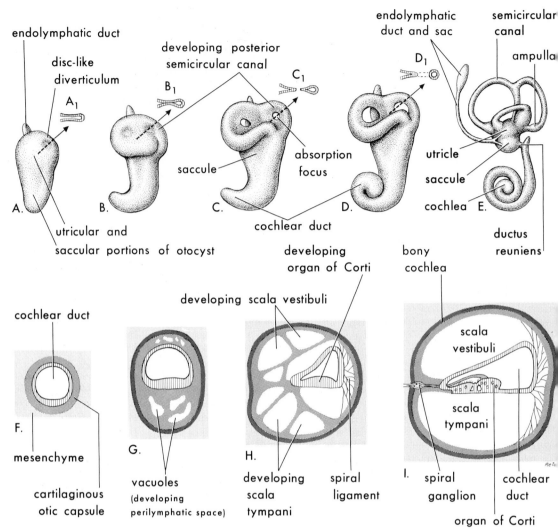

Figure 18–5. Diagrams showing development of the membranous and bony labyrinths of the internal ear. *A* to *E,* Lateral views showing successive stages in the development of the otocyst into the membranous labyrinth from the fifth to eighth weeks. *A₁* to *D₁,* Diagrammatic sketches illustrating the development of a semicircular canal. *F* to *I,* Sections through the cochlear duct showing successive stages in the development of the organ of Corti and the perilymphatic space from the eighth to the twentieth weeks.

fluid, the *perilymph,* in the perilymphatic space. The perilymphatic space related to the cochlear duct develops in two divisions, the *scala tympani* and the *scala vestibuli* (Fig. 18–5H and I). The cartilaginous otic capsule ossifies to form the *bony (osseous) labyrinth* of the internal ear.

The Middle Ear (Fig. 18–6). The tubotympanic recess of the first pharyngeal pouch, described in Chapter 11, expands and becomes the *tympanic cavity.* The unexpanded portion becomes the *pharyngotympanic (Eustachian) tube.*

The External Ear (Figs. 18–6 and 18–7).

The external acoustic meatus develops from the dorsal end of the first branchial groove. The cells at the bottom of this funnel-shaped tube extend inward as a solid epithelial plate called the *meatal plug* (Fig. 18–6C). Late in the fetal period, the central cells of this plug degenerate, forming a cavity which becomes the inner part of the external acoustic meatus.

The early *tympanic membrane* forms from the first branchial or closing membrane (Fig. 18–6A). As development proceeds, mesenchyme extends between the closing membrane and differentiates into the fi-

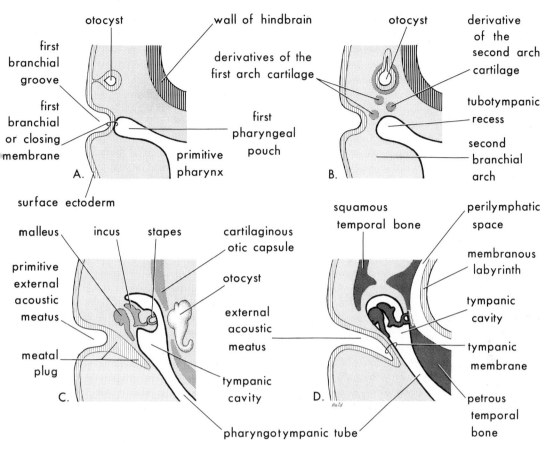

Figure 18–6. Schematic drawings showing development of the middle ear. *A,* Four weeks, illustrating the relation of the otocyst to the branchial apparatus. *B,* Five weeks, showing the tubotympanic recess and branchial arch cartilages. *C,* Later stage, showing the tubotympanic recess (future tympanic cavity) beginning to envelop the ossicles. *D,* Final stage of ear development, showing the relationship of the middle ear to the perilymphatic space and the external acoustic meatus.

brous stratum of the tympanic membrane.

The *auricle* develops from six swellings, called *auricular hillocks,* which develop around the first branchial groove (Fig. 18–7A). As the mandible develops, the ears ascend to the level of the eyes (Fig. 18–7B to D).

CONGENITAL MALFORMATIONS OF THE EYE AND THE EAR

Eye Abnormalities

The critical period of human eye development is from about 24 to 40 days after fertilization. Most congenital abnormalities of the eye appear to be caused by genetic factors or intrauterine infections.

Congenital Cataract. The lens is opaque and frequently appears grayish-white in this condition (see Fig. 9–15A). Many lens opacities are inherited, but some are caused by noxious agents which affect early lens development. Congenital cataract is likely to follow maternal rubella infections which occur during the fourth to sixth weeks when the lens is developing (see Chapter 9).

Cyclopia. In this very rare condition, the eyes are partially or completely fused into a single median eye enclosed in a single orbit. Usually there is a tubular nose (proboscis) above the single eye. The abnormality is frequently associated with other severe malformations which are incompatible with life.

auricular hillocks derived from the first and second branchial arches

A.

first branchial groove

B.

C.

D.

Figure 18–7. Drawings illustrating development of the auricle. *A,* Five weeks. *B,* Six weeks. *C,* Eight weeks. *D,* 32 weeks. As the ears develop, they move from the neck to the side of the head.

Ear Abnormalities

Congenital Deafness. Congenital impairment of hearing may be the result of maldevelopment of the sound-conducting apparatus of the middle ear, or of the neurosensory or perceptive structures of the inner ear. Most types of congenital deafness are caused by autosomal recessive genes. Maternal *rubella infection* during the critical period of development of the ear can cause maldevelopment of the organ of Corti.

Congenital fixation of the stapes results in severe congenital conductive deafness in an otherwise normal ear. Defects of two of the middle ear bones (malleus and incus) are often associated with abnormalities of the first branchial arch (discussed in Chapter 11).

Auricular Abnormalities. There is a wide normal variation in the shape of the auricle. Minor variations are not classified as malformations. The external ears are often abnormal in shape and low-set in malformed infants, especially in chromosomal syndromes (see Table 9–1).

Auricular appendages or tags (Fig. 18–8) in front of the ear are relatively common and result from the development of accessory auricular hillocks.

Atresia of the External Acoustic Meatus. Closure of the meatus results from failure of the meatal plug to canalize. Most cases are associated with the first arch syndrome (see Chapter 11).

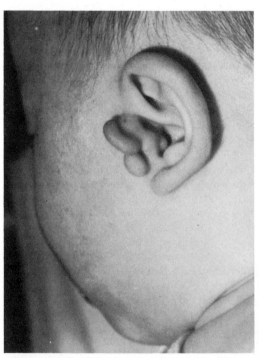

Figure 18–8. Photograph of a child with two auricular appendages or tags. (From Swenson, O.: *Pediatric Surgery.* 1958. Courtesy of Appleton-Century-Crofts, Inc.)

SUMMARY

The eyes and the ears begin to develop during the fourth week. These special sense organs are very sensitive to teratogenic agents, especially viral infections. The most serious defects result from disturbances of development during the fourth to sixth weeks, but defects of sight and hearing may result from developmental disturbances by certain microorganisms during the fetal period.

The Eye. The retina, the optic nerve fibers, the iris muscles, and the epithelium of the iris and ciliary body are derived from the neuroectoderm. The surface ectoderm forms the lens and the epithelium of the lacrimal glands and ducts, the eyelids, the conjunctiva and the cornea. The mesoderm gives rise to the eye muscles (except those of the iris) and all connective and vascular tissues of the cornea, iris, ciliary body, choroid and sclera.

There are many congenital ocular abnormalities, but most of them are rare. Some malformations are caused by defective closure of the optic fissure. Congenital cataract and glaucoma may result from intrauterine rubella infections.

The Ear. The surface ectoderm gives rise to the otocyst which becomes the membranous labyrinth of the internal ear. The body labyrinth develops from the surrounding mesenchyme. The epithelium lining the tympanic cavity, the tympanic antrum, the mastoid air cells and the pharyngotympanic tube is derived from endoderm of the tubotympanic recess of the first pharyngeal pouch. The middle ear bones develop from the cartilages of the first two branchial arches. The external acoustic meatus develops from ectoderm of the first branchial groove (cleft). The tympanic membrane develops from endoderm of the first pharyngeal pouch, from ectoderm of the first branchial groove and from mesenchyme between these layers. The auricle develops from six auricular hillocks or swellings around the first branchial groove.

Congenital deafness may result from abnormal development of the membranous labyrinth or the bony labyrinth or both, as well as from abnormalities of the ossicles. Recessive inheritance is the most common cause of congenital deafness, but prenatal rubella virus infection is a major environmental factor known to cause defective hearing. There are many minor anomalies of the auricle. Low-set malformed ears are often associated with chromosomal abnormalities.

19

THE SKIN, CUTANEOUS APPENDAGES AND TEETH

SKIN

The epidermis is derived from surface ectoderm and the dermis from the mesenchyme under it (Fig. 19–1).

Epidermis. The surface ectodermal cells proliferate and form a protective layer, the *periderm* (Fig. 19–1*B*). Cells from this layer slough off and form part of the *vernix caseosa*, a cheese-like protective substance that covers the skin. By about 11 weeks, cells from the basal layer, or stratum germinativum, have formed an intermediate layer (Fig. 19–1*C*). All layers of the adult epidermis are present at birth (Fig. 19–1*D*).

During the early fetal period, neural crest cells (see Chapter 17) migrate into the dermis and differentiate into *melanoblasts* (Fig. 19–1*C*). These cells soon enter the epidermis and differentiate into *melanocytes* which lie at the epidermal-dermal junction (Fig. 19–1*D*). The melanocytes produce melanin and distribute it to the epidermal cells after birth.

Dermis. The dermis is derived from the mesenchyme underlying the surface ectoderm (Fig. 19–1*A*). By 11 weeks, the mesenchymal cells have begun to produce collagenous and elastic connective tissue fibers (Fig. 19–1*C*). The dermis projects upward into the epidermis and forms *dermal papillae*.

Capillary loops develop in some dermal papillae and sensory nerve endings occur in others.

HAIR

A hair follicle begins as a solid downgrowth of the epidermis into the underlying dermis (Fig. 19–2*A*). The deepest part of the *hair bud* soon becomes club-shaped to form a *hair bulb* (Fig. 19–2*B*). The epithelial cells of the hair bulb constitute the *germinal matrix* which later gives rise to the hair. The hair bulb is then invaginated by a small mesenchymal *hair papilla* (Fig. 19–2*C*). The peripheral cells of the developing hair follicle form the *epithelial root sheath*. The surrounding mesenchymal cells differentiate into the *dermal (connective tissue) root sheath* (Fig. 19–2*D*). As the cells in the *germinal matrix* proliferate, they are pushed upward and become keratinized to form the *hair shaft* (Fig. 19–2*C*). The hair grows, pierces the epidermis and protrudes above the surface of the skin.

Sebaceous Glands

These glands develop as buds from the side of the developing hair follicle (Fig. 19–

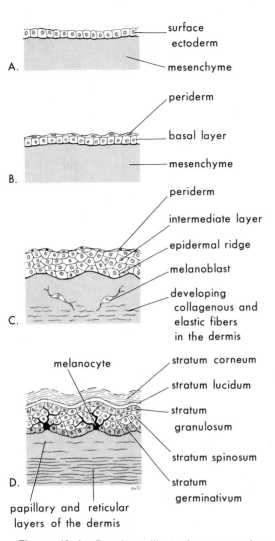

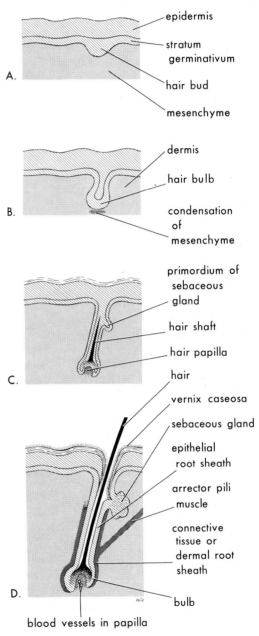

surface
ectoderm

A.

mesenchyme

periderm

basal layer

mesenchyme

B.

periderm

intermediate layer

epidermal ridge

melanoblast

developing
collagenous and
elastic fibers
in the dermis

C.

melanocyte

stratum corneum

stratum lucidum

stratum
granulosum

stratum spinosum

stratum
germinativum

D.

papillary and reticular
layers of the dermis

Figure 19–1. Drawings illustrating successive stages in the development of thick skin. *A*, Four weeks. *B*, Seven weeks. *C*, 11 weeks. *D*, Newborn.

2*C*). The glandular buds grow into the surrounding connective tissue and branch to form the primordia of several alveoli and their associated ducts (Fig. 19–2*D*).

Sweat Glands

These glands develop as solid epidermal downgrowths into the underlying dermis (Fig. 19–3). As the bud elongates, its end becomes coiled to form the primordium of the secretory portion of the gland. The epithelial attachment of the developing gland to the epidermis forms the primordium of the duct.

Nails

The nails begin to develop at about 10 weeks. Development of fingernails precedes that of toenails. The nails first appear as thickened areas of epidermis on the dorsal aspect of each digit (Fig. 19–4*A*). These *nail*

epidermis

stratum
germinativum

A.

hair bud

mesenchyme

dermis

hair bulb

B.

condensation
of
mesenchyme

primordium of
sebaceous
gland

hair shaft

hair papilla

C.

hair

vernix caseosa

sebaceous gland

epithelial
root sheath

arrector pili
muscle

connective
tissue or
dermal root
sheath

D.

bulb

blood vessels in papilla

Figure 19–2. Drawings showing successive stages in the development of a hair and its associated sebaceous gland. *A*, 12 weeks. *B*, 14 weeks. *C*, 16 weeks. *D*, 18 weeks.

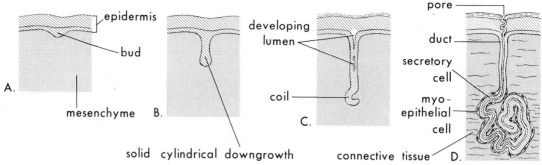

Figure 19–3. Diagrams illustrating successive stages in the development of a sweat gland.

fields are surrounded laterally and proximally by folds of epidermis called *nail folds*. Cells from the proximal nail fold grow over the nail field and become keratinized to form the *nail* or *nail plate* (Fig. 19–4B and C).

MAMMARY GLANDS

The mammary glands develop as solid downgrowths of the epidermis into the underlying mesenchyme (Fig. 19–5C). These occur along two thickened strips of ectoderm, the *mammary ridges* (Fig. 19–5A). Each mammary bud soon gives rise to several secondary buds which develop into *lactiferous ducts* and their branches (Fig. 19–5D and E). The epidermis at the origin of the mammary gland becomes depressed to form a shallow *mammary pit* (Fig. 19–5E). The mammary glands of newborn males and females are often enlarged and some secretion (called "witch's milk") may be produced. These transitory changes are caused by maternal hormones passing into the fetal circulation via the placenta (see Chapter 8).

TEETH

The teeth develop from ectoderm and mesoderm. The enamel is derived from ectoderm of the oral cavity; all other tissues differentiate from mesenchyme.

The Dental Lamina and the Bud Stage. Tooth development begins early in the sixth week as linear U-shaped bands of oral epithelium, called *dental laminae* (Fig. 19–6A). Localized proliferations of cells in the dental laminae produce round or oval swellings called *tooth buds* (Fig. 19–6B). These buds grow into the mesenchyme and develop into the deciduous teeth. The first teeth are called deciduous teeth because they are shed during childhood. There are 10 tooth buds in each jaw, one for each deciduous ("milk") tooth. The tooth buds for the permanent teeth with deciduous predecessors begin to appear at about 10 weeks (Fig. 19–6D).

The Cap Stage. The tooth bud becomes slightly invaginated by mesenchyme called the *dental papilla* (Fig. 19–6C). The dental papilla gives rise to the *dentin* and the *dental pulp*. The developing tooth, called an *enamel*

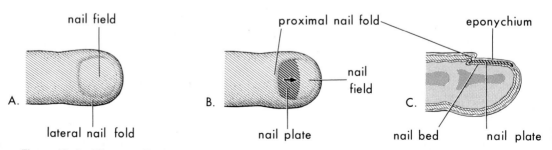

Figure 19–4. Diagrams illustrating successive stages in the development of a fingernail.

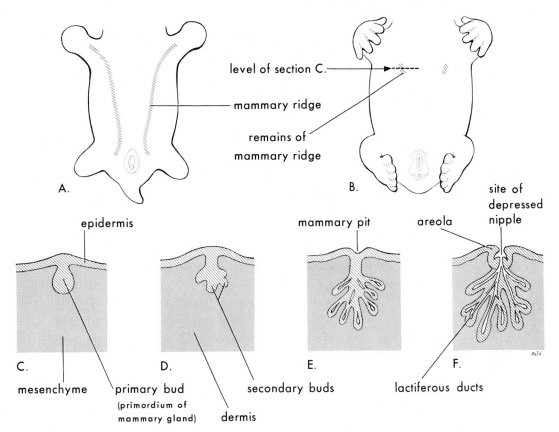

Figure 19–5. Drawings illustrating development of the mammary glands. *A*, Ventral view of an embryo of about 28 days showing the mammary ridges. *B*, Similar view at six weeks showing the remains of these ridges. *C*, Transverse section through the mammary ridge at the site of a developing mammary gland. *D, E* and *F*, Similar sections showing successive stages of development between the twelfth week and birth.

organ, later produces enamel. As the enamel organ and the dental papilla form, the mesenchyme surrounding them condenses and forms a capsule-like structure called the *dental sac* or follicle (Fig. 19–6*E* and *F*). It gives rise to the cementum and the periodontal ligament.

The Bell Stage. As invagination of the enamel organ continues, the developing tooth assumes a bell shape (Fig. 19–6*D*). Mesenchymal cells in the dental papilla adjacent to the inner enamel epithelium differentiate into *odontoblasts*. These cells produce *predentin* and deposit it adjacent to the inner enamel epithelium. Later the predentin calcifies and becomes *dentin*. As the dentin thickens, the odontoblasts regress toward the center of the dental papilla, but processes of the odontoblasts, called *odontoblastic processes*, remain embedded in the dentin (Fig. 19–6*F* and *I*). Cells adjacent to

the dentin differentiate into *ameloblasts*. These cells produce enamel prisms (rods) over the dentin (Fig. 19–6*I*). As the enamel increases, the ameloblasts regress toward the outer enamel epithelium. The inner cells of the dental sac differentiate into *cementoblasts* and produce cementum which is deposited over the dentin of the root.

As the teeth develop and the jaws ossify, the outer cells of the dental sac also become active in bone formation. Each tooth soon becomes surrounded by bone, except over its crown. The tooth is held in its bony socket or *alveolus* by the *periodontal ligament*, a derivative of the dental sac (Fig. 19–6*G*). Some fibers of this ligament are embedded in the cementum, others in the bony wall of the socket.

Tooth Eruption. As the root grows, the crown gradually erupts through the oral mucosa. Eruption of the deciduous teeth

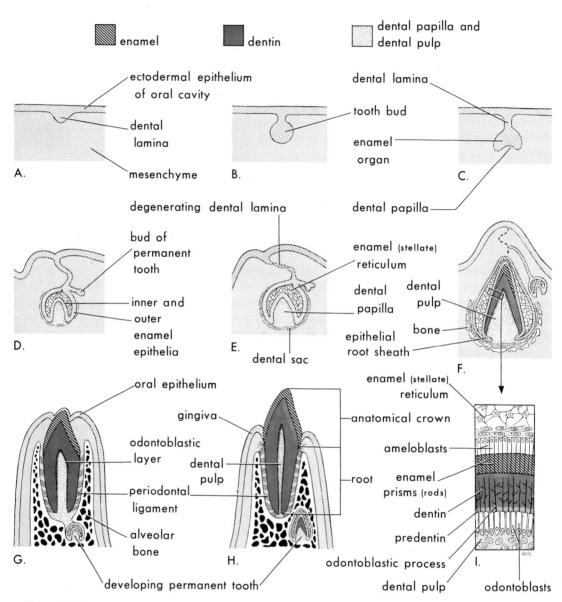

Figure 19–6. Schematic drawings from sagittal sections showing successive stages in the development and eruption of an incisor tooth. *A,* Six weeks, showing the dental lamina. *B,* Seven weeks, showing the bud stage of tooth development. *C,* Eight weeks, showing the cap stage of development of the enamel organ. *D,* 10 weeks, showing the early bell stage of the enamel organ of the deciduous tooth and the bud stage of the developing permanent tooth. *E,* 14 weeks, showing the advanced bell stage of the enamel organ. Note that the connection (dental lamina) of the tooth to the oral epithelium is degenerating. *F,* 28 weeks, showing the enamel and dentin layers. *G,* Six months *postnatal,* showing early tooth eruption. *H,* 18 months *postnatal,* showing a fully erupted deciduous incisor tooth. The permanent incisor tooth now has a well developed crown. *I,* Section through a developing tooth showing the ameloblasts (enamel producers) and the odontoblasts (dentin producers).

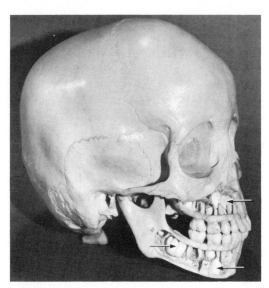

Figure 19–7. Photograph of the skull of a child in the fourth year. The jaws have been dissected to show the relations of the developing permanent teeth (arrows) to the deciduous teeth.

usually occurs between the sixth and twenty-fourth month after birth.

The permanent teeth develop in a manner similar to that previously described for deciduous teeth (Fig. 19–7). As a permanent tooth grows, the root of the corresponding deciduous tooth is gradually resorbed by osteoclasts. Consequently, when the deciduous tooth is shed it consists only of the crown and the uppermost portion of the root. The permanent teeth usually begin to erupt during the sixth year and continue to appear until early adulthood.

CONGENITAL MALFORMATIONS

Congenital Alopecia (Atrichia Congenita). Fetal absence or loss of hair may occur alone or with other abnormalities of the skin and its derivatives. The hair loss may be caused by failure of hair follicles to develop or result from follicles producing poor-quality hairs.

Hypertrichosis. Excessive hairiness results from the development of excess hair follicles or from the persistence of hairs that normally disappear during the fetal period. Localized hypertrichosis is often associated with spina bifida occulta (see Chapter 17).

Supernumerary Breasts and Nipples (Fig. 19–8). An extra breast (*polymastia*) occurs in about one per cent of the female population and is an inheritable condition. Supernumerary nipples (*polythelia*) are also relatively common and they may also occur in males. An extra breast or nipple usually develops just below the normal breast. In these positions, the extra nipples or breasts develop from extra mammary buds along the mammary ridges. Accessory breasts may have normal breast tissue and become functional during pregnancy.

Enamel Hypoplasia. Defective enamel formation results in grooves, pits (Fig. 19–9*B*) or fissures on the enamel surface. These conditions result from a temporary disturbance in enamel formation. Various factors may injure the ameloblasts (e. g., tetracycline therapy and diseases such as measles).

Abnormalities in Shape (Fig. 19–9*A* to *G*). Abnormally shaped teeth are relatively common. Occasionally, spherical masses of enamel, called *enamel pearls*, are attached to the tooth (Fig. 19–9*B*). They are formed by aberrant groups of ameloblasts.

Numerical Abnormalities (Fig. 19–9*H* and *I*). One or more supernumerary teeth may develop, or teeth may not form.

Fused Teeth (Fig. 19–8*C* and *G*). Occasionally, a tooth bud divides or two buds partially fuse to form fused or joined teeth. In some cases the permanent tooth does not form.

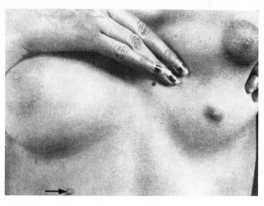

Figure 19–8. Photograph of an adult female with a supernumerary nipple on the right (arrow) and a supernumerary breast below the normal left one. (From Haagensen, C. D.: *Diseases of the Breast*, 2nd Ed. 1971. Courtesy of the W. B. Saunders Company.)

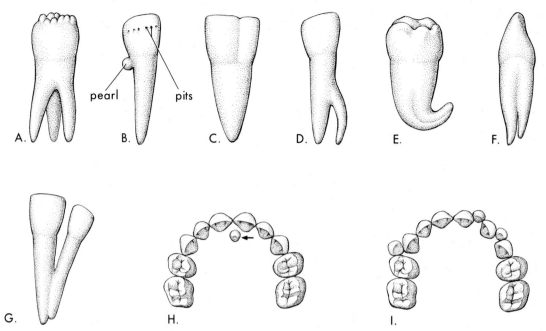

Figure 19–9. Drawings illustrating abnormalities of teeth. *A,* Irregular raspberry-like crown. *B,* Enamel pearl and pits. *C,* Incisor tooth with a double crown. *D,* Abnormal division of root. *E,* Distorted root. *F,* Branched root. *G,* Fused roots. *H,* Hyperdontia, with a supernumerary incisor tooth in the anterior region of the palate (arrow). *I,* Hyperdontia, with 13 deciduous teeth in the upper jaw instead of the normal 10.

SUMMARY

The epidermis and its derivatives (hairs, nails and glands) are derived from surface ectoderm. Hairs develop from downgrowths of the epidermis into the dermis. The sebaceous glands develop as outgrowths from the side of hair follicles. The sweat and mammary glands develop from epidermal downgrowths. Supernumerary breasts (polymastia) or nipples (polythelia) are relatively common.

The teeth develop from ectoderm and mesoderm. The enamel is produced by cells derived from ectoderm; all other dental tissues develop from mesoderm. The common congenital malformations of teeth are defective formation of enamel and dentin, abnormalities in shape and variations in number and position.

REFERENCES

Recommended Books for Further Reading

Hamilton, W. J., Boyd, J. D., and Mossman, H. W.: *Human Embryology. Prenatal Development of Form and Function*. 4th Ed. Cambridge, W. Heffer and Sons, Ltd., 1972.
Langman, J.: *Medical Embryology*. 2nd Ed. Baltimore, The Williams & Wilkins Co., 1969.
Moore, K. L.: *The Developing Human. Clinically Oriented Embryology*. Philadelphia, W. B. Saunders Co., 1973.
Patten, B. M.: *Human Embryology*. 3rd Ed. New York, The Blakiston Division, McGraw-Hill Book Co., 1968.
Rugh, R., and Shettles, L. B.: *From Conception to Birth. The Drama of Life's Beginnings*. New York, Harper & Row, 1971.

Chapter 1

Arey, L. B.: *Developmental Anatomy: A Textbook and Laboratory Manual of Embryology*. 7th Ed. Philadelphia, W. B. Saunders Co., 1965, pp. 1–6.
Meyer, A. W.: *The Rise of Embryology*. Stanford, Cal., Stanford University Press, 1939.
Needham, J.: *A History of Embryology*. 2nd Ed. Cambridge, Cambridge University Press, 1959.
Streeter, G. L.: Developmental horizons in human embryos: Description of age group XI, 13 to 20 somites, and age group XII, 21 to 29 somites. *Contr. Embryol. Carneg. Instn. 30*:211, 1942.
Willis, R. A.: *The Borderland of Embryology and Pathology*. 2nd Ed. London, Butterworth & Co. (Publishers), Ltd., 1962.

Chapter 2

Böving, B.: Anatomy of reproduction; *in* J. P. Greenhill (ed.): *Obstetrics*. 13th Ed. Philadelphia, W. B. Saunders Co., 1965, pp. 1–101.
Brown, R. L.: Rate of transport of sperma in the human uterus and the tubes. *Amer. J. Obstet. Gynec. 47*:153, 1955.
Gamzell, C.: Ovulation; *in* E. E. Philipp, J. Barnes, and M. Newton (eds.): *Scientific Foundations of Obstetrics and Gynecology*. London, William Heinemann, Ltd., 1970, pp. 131–134.
Hancock, J. L.: The sperm cell. *Science J.* (London) *6*:31, 1970.
Klopper, A.: The reproductive hormones. *Science J.* (London) *6*:44, 1970.
Leeson, T. S., and Leeson, C. R.: *Histology*. 2nd Ed. Philadelphia, W. B. Saunders Co., 1970, pp. 416–462.

Chapter 3

Allen, R. C.: The moment of fertilization. *Sci. Amer. 201*:124, 1959.
Austin, C. R.: The egg and fertilization. *Science J.* (London) *6*:37, 1970.
Edwards, R. G., and Fowler, R. E.: Human embryos in the laboratory. *Sci. Amer. 223*:44, 1970.
Gilbert, M. S.: *Biography of the Newborn*. New York, Hafner Publishing Co., Inc., 1963.
Hertig, A. T., and Rock, J.: Two human ova of the pre-villous stage, having a developmental age of about seven and nine days respectively. *Contr. Embryol. Carneg. Instn. 31*:65, 1945.
Shettles, L. B.: *Ovum Humanum*. New York, Hafner Publishing Co., Inc., 1960.

Chapter 4

Benirschke, K.: Implantation, placental development, uteroplacental blood flow; *in* D. E. Reid, K. J. Ryan, and K. Benirschke: *Principles and Management of Human Reproduction*. Philadelphia, W. B. Saunders Co., 1972, pp. 179–196.
Boronow, R. C., McElin, T. W., West, R. H., and Buckingham, J. C.: Ovarian Pregnancy. *Amer. J. Obstet. Gynec. 91*:1095, 1965.
Carr, D. H.: Chromosome anomalies as a cause of spontaneous abortion. *Amer. J. Obstet. Gynec. 97*:283, 1967.

Hertig, A. T., and Rock, J.: Two human ova of the pre-villous stage, having a developmental age of about eleven and twelve days respectively. *Contr. Embryol. Carneg. Instn. 29*:127, 1941.
Reid, D. E., and Benirschke, K.: Ectopic pregnancy; *in* D. E. Reid, K. J. Ryan, and K. Benirschke: *Principles and Management of Human Reproduction.* Philadelphia, W. B. Saunders Co., 1972, pp. 277–285.
Stander, R. W.: Abdominal pregnancy. *Clin. Obstet. Gynec. 5*:1065, 1962.

Chapter 5

Bessis, M.: The blood cells and their formation; *in* J. Brachet and A. E. Mirsky (eds.): *The Cell.* Vol. 5. New York, Academic Press, 1961, pp. 163–217.
Hamilton, W. J., and Boyd, J. D.: Development of the human placenta; *in* E. E. Philipp, J. Barnes, and M. Newton (eds.): *Scientific Foundations of Obstetrics and Gynecology.* London, William Heinemann, Ltd., 1970, pp. 185–254.
Jones, H. O., and Brewer, J. I.: A human ovum in the primitive streak stage. *Contr. Embryol. Carneg. Instn. 29*:157, 1941.
Wide, L.: Immunological determination of human gonadotrophins: *in* E. E. Philipp, J. Barnes, and M. Newton (eds.): *Scientific Foundations of Obstetrics and Gynecology.* London, William Heinemann Ltd., 1970, pp. 509–514.
Wilson, K. M.: A normal human ovum of 16 days development, the Rochester ovum. *Contr. Embryol. Carneg. Instn. 31*:103, 1945.

Chapter 6

Langman, J.: *Medical Embryology: Human Development—Normal and Abnormal.* 2nd Ed. Baltimore, The Williams & Wilkins Co., 1969, pp. 107–126.
Nishimura, H., Takano, K., Tanimura, T., and Yasuda, M.: Normal and abnormal development of human embryos. *Teratology 1*:281, 1968.
Shepard, T. H.: Normal and abnormal growth patterns; *in* L. I. Gardner (ed.): *Endocrine and Genetic Diseases of Childhood.* Philadelphia, W. B. Saunders Co., 1969, pp. 1–6.
Streeter, G. L.: Developmental horizons in human embryos: Description of age group XIII, embryos of 4 or 5 millimeters long, and age group XIV, period of identification of the lens vesicle. *Contr. Embryol. Carneg. Instn. 31*:27, 1945.
Yamada, T.: Factors of Embryonic induction; *in* M. Florkin and E. H. Stotz (eds.): *Comprehensive Biochemistry.* Vol. 28. Amsterdam, Elsevier Publishing Co., 1967.

Chapter 7

Gruenwald, P.: Growth of the human fetus. I. Normal growth and its variation. *Amer. J. Obstet. Gynec. 94*:1112, 1966.
Hellman, L. M., Kobayashi, M., Fillisti, L., and Cromb, E.: The sonographic depiction of the growth and development of the human fetus; *in* R. Caldeyro-Barcia (ed.): *Perinatal Factors Affecting Human Development.* Washington, D. C., Pan American Health Organization, Scientific Publication No. 185, 1969, pp. 70–80.
Liley, A. W.: The use of amniocentesis and fetal transfusion in erythroblastosis fetalis. *Pediatrics 35*:876, 1965.
Moore, K. L.: *The Sex Chromatin.* Philadelphia, W. B. Saunders Co., 1966, pp. 1–6.
Nyhan, W. L.: Intra-uterine diagnosis and the antenatal detection of inherited disease; *in* P. Benson (ed.): *The Biochemistry of Development.* London, William Heinemann, Ltd., 1971, pp. 14–29.
Shepard, T. H.: Normal and abnormal growth patterns; *in* L. I. Gardner (ed.): *Endocrine and Genetic Diseases of Childhood.* Philadelphia, W. B. Saunders Co., 1969, pp. 1–6.
Streeter, G. L.: Weight, sitting height, head size, foot length and menstrual age of the human embryo. *Contr. Embryol. Carneg. Instn. 11*:143, 1920.

Chapter 8

Allen, F. H., Jr., and Umansky, I.: Erythroblastosis fetalis; *in* D. E. Reid, K. J. Ryan, and K. Benirschke: *Principles and Management of Human Reproduction.* Philadelphia, W. B. Saunders Co., 1972, pp. 811–832.
Benirschke, K., and Driscoll, S. G.: *The Pathology of the Human Placenta.* New York, Springer-Verlag, 1967.
Benirschke, K., and Reid, D. E.: Multiple pregnancy; *in* D. E. Reid, K. J. Ryan, and K. Benirschke: *Principles and Management of Human Reproduction.* Philadelphia, W. B. Saunders Co., 1972, pp. 197–210.
Boyd, J. D., and Hamilton, W. J.: *The Human Placenta.* Cambridge, W. Heffer & Sons, Ltd., 1970.

Bulmer, M. G.: *The Biology of Twinning in Man.* Oxford, The Clarendon Press, 1970.

Javert, C. T.: *Spontaneous and Habitual Abortion.* New York, The Blakiston Division, McGraw-Hill Book Co., 1957.

Torpin, R.: *The Human Placenta.* Springfield, Ill., Charles C Thomas, Publisher, 1969.

Villee, C. A. (ed.): *The Placenta and Fetal Membranes.* Baltimore, The Williams & Wilkins Co., 1960.

Chapter 9

Bartalos, M., and Baramki, T. A.: *Medical Cytogenetics.* Baltimore, The Williams & Wilkins Co., 1967.

Berlin, C. M., and Jacobson, C. B.: Congenital anomalies associated with parental LSD ingestion. *Society for Pediatric Research Abstracts. Second Plenary Session,* 1970.

Breg, W. R.: Autosomal abnormalities; *in* L. I. Gardner (ed.): *Endocrine and Genetic Diseases of Childhood.* Philadelphia, W. B. Saunders Co., 1969, pp. 608–631.

Carter, C. O.: The genetics of congenital malformations; *in* E. E. Philipp, J. Barnes, and M. Newton (eds.): *Scientific Foundations of Obstetrics and Gynecology.* London, William Heinemann, Ltd., 1970, pp. 665–670.

Ferguson-Smith, M. A.: Sex Chromatin, Klinefelter's syndrome and mental deficiency; *in* Moore, K. L. (ed.): *The Sex Chromatin.* Philadelphia, W. B. Saunders Co., 1966, pp. 277–315.

Fraser, F. C.: Etiologic agents. II. Physical and chemical agents; *in* A. Rubin (ed.): *Handbook of Congenital Malformations.* Philadelphia, W. B. Saunders Co., 1967, pp. 365–371.

Hicks, S. P., and D'Amato, C. J.: Effects of ionizing radiations on mammalian development. *Advanc. Teratol. 1*:195, 1966.

Karnofsky, D. A.: Drugs as teratogens in animals and man. *Ann. Rev. Pharmacol.* 5:447, 1965.

Moore, K. L.: The vulnerable embryo: Causes of malformation in man. *Manitoba Med. Rev. 43*:306, 1963.

Persaud, T. V. N., and Ellington, A. C.: Teratogenic activity of cannabis resin. *Lancet* 2:406, 1968.

Saxén, L., and Rapola, J.: *Congenital Defects.* New York, Holt, Rinehart & Winston, Inc., 1969, pp. 35–75.

Smith, D. W.: *Recognizable Patterns of Human Malformation: Genetic, Embryologic, and Clinical Aspects.* Philadelphia, W. B. Saunders Co., 1970.

Smithels, R. W.: Drugs and human malformations. *Advanc. Teratol. 1*:251, 1966.

Tuchmann-Duplessis, H.: The effects of teratogenic drugs; *in* E. E. Philipp, J. Barnes, and M. Newton (eds.): *Scientific Foundations of Obstetrics and Gynecology.* London, William Heinemann, Ltd., 1970, pp. 636–648.

Warkany, J.: *Congenital Malformations: Notes and Comments.* Chicago, Year Book Medical Publishers, Inc., 1971.

Chapter 10

Areechon, W., and Reid, L.: Hypoplasia of the lung with congenital diaphragmatic hernia. *Brit. Med. J. 1*:230, 1963.

Butler, N., and Claireaux, A. E.: Congenital diaphragmatic hernia as a cause of perinatal mortality. *Lancet* 1:659, 1962.

Tarnay, T. J.: Diaphragmatic hernia. *Ann. Thorac. Surg.* 5:66, 1968.

Chapter 11

Albers, G. D.: Branchial anomalies. *J.A.M.A. 183*:399, 1963.

Kernahan, D. A., and Stark, R. B.: A new classification for cleft lip and cleft palate. *Plast. Reconstr. Surg. 22*:435, 1958.

MacCollum, D. W., and Rubin, A.: Cleft lip and cleft palate; *in* A. Rubin (ed.): *Handbook of Congenital Malformations.* Philadelphia, W. B. Saunders Co., 1967, pp. 114–117.

Mathews, D. N.: Hare lip and cleft palate; *in* J. C. Mustardé (ed.): *Plastic Surgery in Infancy and Childhood.* Edinburgh, E. & S. Livingstone, Ltd., 1971, pp. 1–36.

Moseley, J. M., Mathews, E. W., Breed, R. H., Galante, E., Tse, A., and MacIntyre, I.: The ultimobranchial origin of calcitonin. *Lancet 1*:108, 1968.

Remnick, H.: *Embryology of the Face and Oral Cavity.* Rutherford, N. J., Fairleigh Dickinson University Press, 1970.

Wilson, C. P.: Lateral cysts and fistulas of the neck of developmental origin. *Ann. Roy. Coll. Surg. Eng. 17*:1, 1955.

Chapter 12

Avery, M. E.: *The Lung and Its Disorders in the Newborn Infant.* 2nd Ed. Philadelphia, W. B. Saunders Co., 1968.

Boyden, E. A.: Development of the human lung; *in* J. Brennemann (ed.): *Practice of Pediatrics*. Vol. IV. Hagerstown, Md., W. F. Prior Co., Inc., 1971.

Emery, J.: *The Anatomy of the Developing Lung*. London, William Heinemann, Ltd., 1969.

Landing, B. H.: Anomalies of the respiratory tract. *Pediat. Clin. N. Amer*. Philadelphia, W. B. Saunders Co., February, 1957.

Salzberg, A. M.: Congenital malformations of the lower respiratory tract; *in* E. L. Kendig (ed.): *Disorders of the Respiratory Tract in Children*. Philadelphia, W. B. Saunders Co., 1967, pp. 493–540.

Smith, E. I.: The early development of the trachea and oesophagus in relation to atresia of the oesophagus and tracheo-oesophageal fistula. *Contr. Embryol. Carneg. Instn. 245*:36, 1957.

Waterson, D. J., Carter, R. E., and Aberdeen, E.: Oesophageal atresia: tracheo-oesophageal fistula, a study of survival in 218 infants. *Lancet 1*:819, 1962.

Chapter 13

Bremer, J. L.: *Congenital Anomalies of the Viscera*. Cambridge, Mass., Harvard University Press, 1957.

Estrada, R. L.: *Anomalies of Intestinal Rotation and Fixation*. Springfield, Ill., Charles C Thomas, Publisher, 1968.

Gray, S. W., and Skandalakis, J. E.: *Embryology for Surgeons. The Embryological Basis for the Treatment of Congenital Defects*. Philadelphia, W. B. Saunders Co., 1972, pp. 63–281.

Stephens, F. D.: *Congenital Malformations of the Rectum, Anus and Genito-Urinary Tracts*. Edinburgh, E. & S. Livingstone, Ltd., 1963.

Chapter 14

Federman, D. D.: *Abnormal Sexual Development: A Genetic and Endocrine Approach to Differential Diagnosis*. Philadelphia, W. B. Saunders Co., 1967.

Jones, H. H., and Scott, W. W.: *Hermaphroditism, Genital Anomalies and Related Endocrine Disorders*. Baltimore, The Williams & Wilkins Co., 1958.

Moore, K. L.: Sex determination, sexual differentiation and intersex development. *Canad. Med. Ass. J. 97*:292, 1967.

Schlegel, R. J., and Gardner, L. I.: Ambiguous and abnormal genitalia in infants: differential diagnosis and clinical management; *in* L. I. Gardner (ed.): *Endocrine and Genetic Diseases of Childhood*. Philadelphia, W. B. Saunders Co., 1969, pp. 522–539.

Chapter 15

Anderson, R. C.: Causative factors underlying congenital heart malformations. *Pediatrics 14*:143, 1954.

Campbell, M.: Place of maternal rubella in the aetiology of congenital heart disease. *Brit. Med. J. 1*:691, 1961.

Duckworth, J. W. A.: Embryology of congenital heart disease; *in* J. D. Keith, R. D. Rowe, and P. Vlad (eds.): *Heart Disease in Infancy and Childhood*. 2nd Ed. New York, The Macmillan Co., 1967, pp. 136–158.

Edwards, J. E., Dry, T. J., Parker, R. L., Burchell, H. B., Wood, E. H., and Bulbulian, A. H.: *An Atlas of Congenital Anomalies of the Heart and Great Vessels*. Springfield, Ill., Charles C Thomas, Publisher, 1954.

Mitchell, S. C.: The ductus arteriosus in the neonatal period. *J. Pediat. 51*:12, 1957.

Moss, A. J., and Adams, F. H.: *Heart Disease in Infants, Children and Adolescents*. Baltimore, The Williams & Wilkins Co., 1968.

Chapter 16

Bayer, L. M., and Bayley, N.: *Growth Diagnosis. Selected Methods for Interpreting and Predicting Physical Development From One Year to Maturity*. Chicago, The University of Chicago Press, 1959.

Frantz, C. H., and O'Rahilly, R.: Congenital skeletal limb deficiencies. *J. Bone Joint Surg., 43A*:1202, 1961.

Gasser, R. F.: The development of the facial muscles in man. *Amer. J. Anat. 120*:357, 1967.

Lenz, W., and Knapp, K.: Foetal malformations due to thalidomide. *German Med. Monthly 7*:253, 1962.

Noback, C. R., and Robertson, G. G.: Sequences of appearance of ossification centers in the human skeleton during the first five prenatal months. *Amer. J. Anat. 89*:1, 1951.

Swinyard, C. A. (ed.): *Limb Development and Deformity: Problems of Evaluation and Rehabilitation*. Springfield, Ill., Charles C Thomas, Publisher, 1969.

Chapter 17

Dennison, W. M.: Spina bifida; *in* J. C. Mustardé (ed.): *Plastic Surgery in Infancy and Childhood.* Edinburgh, E. & S. Livingstone, Ltd., 1971, pp. 381–385.

Giroud, A.: Causes and morphogenesis of anencephaly; *in* G. E. W. Wolstenholme and C. M. O'Connor (eds.): *Ciba Foundation Symposium on Congenital Malformations.* London, J. & A. Churchill, 1960, pp. 199–212.

Kalter, H.: *Teratology of the Central Nervous System.* Chicago, University of Chicago Press, 1968.

Laurence, K. M., and Weeks, R.: Abnormalities of the central nervous system; *in* A. P. Norman (ed.): *Congenital Abnormalities in Infancy.* 2nd Ed. Oxford, Blackwell Scientific Publications, 1971, pp. 25–86.

Chapter 18

Brown, C. A.: Abnormalities of the eyes and associated structures; *in* A. P. Norman (ed.): *Congenital Abnormalities in Infancy.* 2nd Ed. Oxford, Blackwell Scientific Publications, 1971, pp. 147–198.

Gray, J. E.: Rubella in pregnancy; fetal pathology in the internal ear. *Ann. Otol. 68*:170, 1959.

Haydon, G. D., and Arnold, G. G.: The ear; *in* E. L. Kendig, Jr. (ed.): *Disorders of the Respiratory Tract in Children.* Philadelphia, W. B. Saunders Co., 1968, pp. 215–240.

Mann, I. C.: *Developmental Abnormalities of the Eye.* 2nd Ed. Philadelphia, J. B. Lippincott Co., 1957.

Sharp, H. S.: Abnormalities of the ear, nose and throat; *in* A. P. Norman (ed.): *Congenital Abnormalities in Infancy.* 2nd Ed. Oxford, Blackwell Scientific Publications, 1971, pp. 131–146.

Willis, N. R., Hollenberg, M. J., and Braekevelt, C. R.: The fine structure of the lens of the fetal rat. *Canad. J. Ophthal. 4*:307, 1969.

Chapter 19

Haagensen, C. D.: *Diseases of the Breast.* 2nd Ed. Philadelphia, W. B. Saunders Co., 1971.

Moynahan, E. J.: Abnormalities of the skin; *in* A. P. Norman (ed.): *Congenital Abnormalities in Infancy.* 2nd Ed. Oxford, Blackwell Scientific Publications, 1971, pp. 289–349.

Shafer, W. G., Hine, M. K., and Levy, B. M.: *A Textbook of Oral Pathology.* 2nd Ed. Philadelphia, W. B. Saunders Co., 1963.

Sicher, H., and Bhaskar, S. N.: *Orban's Oral Histology and Embryology.* 7th Ed. St. Louis, The C. V. Mosby Co., 1972.

INDEX

Note: Page references in *italic* refer to illustrations; those followed by (t) refer to tables.